A Comprehensive Guide for Adult Women Navigating ADHD

Techniques and Skills to Positively Transform Your Life and Take Charge of Adult ADHD

Lillian Clem

© Copyright 2021 - All rights reserved.

The content contained within this book may not be reproduced, duplicated or transmitted without direct written permission from the author or the publisher.

Under no circumstances will any blame or legal responsibility be held against the publisher, or author, for any damages, reparation, or monetary loss due to the information contained within this book, either directly or indirectly.

Legal Notice:

This book is copyright protected. It is only for personal use. You cannot amend, distribute, sell, use, quote or paraphrase any part, or the content within this book, without the consent of the author or publisher.

Disclaimer Notice:

Please note the information contained within this document is for educational and entertainment purposes only. All effort has been executed to present accurate, up to date, reliable, complete information. No warranties of any kind are declared or implied. Readers acknowledge that the author is not engaged in the rendering of legal, financial, medical or professional advice. The content within this book has been derived from various sources. Please consult a licensed professional before attempting any techniques outlined in this book.

By reading this document, the reader agrees that under no circumstances is the author responsible for any losses, direct or indirect, that are incurred as a result of the use of the information contained within this document, including, but not limited to, errors, omissions, or inaccuracies.

Table of Contents

INTRODUCTION 1
   THE CONTENT OF THE BOOK 3

CHAPTER 1: INTRODUCTION TO ADHD 7
   TYPES OF ADHD 7
      How Is ADHD Diagnosed in Adults? 14

CHAPTER 2: HOW ADHD PRESENTS IN WOMEN 27
   DIFFERENCES IN MEN AND WOMEN 27
      Let's Talk About Comorbid Conditions 31

CHAPTER 3: TIPS AND TECHNIQUES TO HELP WOMEN DEAL WITH ADHD 45
   TREATMENT STRATEGIES FOR CO-OCCURRING ADHD AND SUBSTANCE USE DISORDERS 52

CHAPTER 4: DEALING WITH DIFFERENT SITUATIONS AND SETTINGS 63
   DEALING WITH DAILY STRUGGLES IN DIFFERENT ENVIRONMENTS 63
      Homelife 68
   PARENTHOOD 78
   RELATIONSHIPS 84

CHAPTER 5: IMPROVING YOUR FOCUS 89
   GAMES THAT IMPROVE YOUR FOCUS 89
   THE BENEFITS OF EXERCISE 91

CHAPTER 6: INTERESTING FACTS ABOUT THE HISTORY OF ADHD 97
   WHAT THE FUTURE MAY HOLD 99

CHAPTER 7: THE POSITIVE SIDE OF ADHD (SURPRISING STRENGTHS) 103
   SUPERPOWERS 103
   SUPER WOMEN 106

CHAPTER 8: DEBUNKING MYTHS ABOUT ADHD 117
   THE MOST COMMON MYTHS 117
   WHY IT'S IMPORTANT TO SPREAD AWARENESS 119

CHAPTER 9: SELF-CARE 121
   SELF-CARE IDEAS 121

CHAPTER 10: EMBRACE WHO YOU ARE, ACCEPT YOURSELF.............. 125
- Newly Diagnosed as an Adult Woman... 126

CHAPTER 11: DECISION-MAKING.. 131
- Tips on How to Take Charge of Your Decisions................................. 131
  - *Sticking to Your Choices.. 136*

CHAPTER 12: MANAGING YOUR FINANCES.. 139
- Budgeting... 139

CHAPTER 13: SOCIAL GATHERINGS.. 145
- Tips on How to Host and Plan Without Unnecessary Stress!.......... 145
- Meal Planning... 147
- Easy Meals.. 149

CONCLUSION.. 163
- You're Not Alone!... 163

REFERENCES.. 167

Introduction

"Life could be a dream, if I could take you up in paradise up above."
- The Coasters

What if life could be a dream? What if things didn't have to be so hard all the time? If we could just learn to love ourselves the way we are, instead of criticizing ourselves for every wrong step?

When they sing, "If you could tell me that I'm the only one that you love," what if this could be a love song directed at yourself, instead?

I'm not a doctor, I'm not an expert who spent years studying the effects of and treatments that were developed for ADHD. I'm simply a woman who's spent her life locked in a brawl with her own mind. I spent years looking for answers, a way to live a normal life.

It was when I was at my lowest that I decided that I needed to stand up for myself and, most importantly, accept myself. See, our brains work differently, some parts are underactive or overactive. We have less dopamine and other chemicals than most people, and a rare group of us seem to have more.

We are stronger than the world gives us credit for; along with the battles that every woman faces in this life, we also battle our own internal turmoil in the form of Attention Deficit Hyperactivity Disorder. We also fight overwhelming emotions and intense feelings of failure. We fight an inability to focus, and we fight alone...

Here's the thing... we're not alone! You are *not alone*! There are thousands if not millions of women who have the same condition as you do. The symptoms might not be 100% the same, but they are similar enough for us to be able to relate to them and to each other.

Do you want to take control of your life? The power is within you! Yes, I know, totally cliché. But it's the truth. I spent so much time researching and observing and learning, I felt like every doctor was saying the same thing. Try this or try that, here's a pill. It felt like an endless cycle.

Until I realized that this is my brain, this is my life, this is my future *and I control it*. I decided to write this book to educate women on ADHD but also to offer some advice that I've found to be helpful.

During my journey, I have realized that it is actually pretty helpful to listen to your doctor. When you understand where they're coming from, how it all started, and what kinds of advances we've had in treatments in recent years, you begin to understand how important their advice is.

When you understand why certain medications work, you begin to understand that it's not just simply a pill. But most importantly, you realize that even though you are a strong and brave woman who is capable of anything, you do sometimes need a little help.

Controlling your life and your future doesn't mean that you go off the grid and sip herbal teas instead of listening to the professionals, though herbal teas do have many health benefits. It means that you make a conscious decision to change your life and be the best that you can be. You do this by taking care of yourself, and that includes letting the experts help you!

This book is for every woman with ADHD who is tired or nearing their breaking point. It's also for those who want to understand what it's like to live with this condition in order to better support a loved one.

I've read so many fantastic books on the subject, but they were all written by doctors. While this is an incredibly helpful perspective, I yearned for true understanding. I'm sure that there must be other books written by women with ADHD out there, I've just not found them. That's why I decided to write this book, to try and connect with all the superwomen who hold themselves together despite these challenges every day.

Sometimes, it's nice to hear from someone who truly feels what you feel, who has been in many of the situations you have. For this reason, I'm here today.

The Content of the Book

Here's what can be expected. Like most books that revolve around mental health conditions or other conditions, we need to look at the clinical definition and the facts first. I want every person who reads this book to walk away with a comprehensive understanding of their condition without having to consult Google every five minutes. That's what chapter one will essentially be, an introduction to ADHD. I'll also be discussing different types of ADHD and how diagnosis takes place.

In chapter two, we'll take a look at how ADHD presents in women specifically and what the differences between men and women with the condition are. For example, men tend to be more socially disruptive and women tend to be more inattentive. It used to be thought that ADHD was more commonly diagnosed in men. This has been debunked as a myth. Women simply experience their symptoms differently.

Chapter three will have all kinds of tips for dealing with daily struggles that we face. When you understand what some of those are, you can start working through them. We'll be covering tips for time management and avoiding procrastination, as these are important for our future and success. You can also expect to learn some problem-solving skills to avoid any extra frustration, since that seems to be an old friend of ours. This will also include treatment strategies for co-occurring ADHD and SUD.

Chapter four will offer advice on how to deal with difficult situations that may arise within certain settings such as your workplace. I'll also be advising on home life and your social life; sometimes all we need is a breather. What better way to do that than in an organized home! As women with ADHD, I'm sure that most of you understand the frustrations that can come with disorganization and clutter.

You probably also understand that procrastination and a lack of motivation can keep us from doing something about it. Whether you're a young woman living in her first apartment with a cat and a bunch of plant babies, a married woman with children, or an older woman living by herself or with a partner, your house needs cleaning at some point. Women with ADHD can often have trouble with this aspect of home life. After your declutter and organizational adventure, you'll need to still regularly clean your home. Simply keeping it organized is not enough! So, I will also be giving some tips on how to create a cleaning schedule with a checklist and a few quick cleaning tips.

Chapter five will offer some extra advice on how to improve and maintain your focus. Brain games, calming techniques, and exercise all benefit you! Chapter six is all about where it all began, some interesting facts about the history of ADHD and the first forms of treatment. Researching the topic has definitely made me thankful for the advances in medicine and technology!

Now that we've had an extensive look at the condition and how to deal with or treat symptoms, it's safe to say that it would be time to look at the bright side. People with ADHD sometimes have surprising strengths and talents. Our condition is not a death sentence! It's a part of who we are and it makes us unique. Chapter seven will go into more detail about the facts mentioned above.

On that note, there are so many myths and stigmas that surround ADHD. Some of them are outright appalling. For this reason, I've decided to debunk some of the most common ones here. We face enough, I'm pretty sure that most of us could do without them, and for those reading this in support of a loved one, some clarification should help your mission. Chapter eight will be all about these myths and stigmas.

Chapter nine will explore some options for self-care. Let's face it, any woman needs the right amount of self-care. Even if it's something as simple as taking a 15-minute break or having a glass of wine after a long day. When you constantly battle for survival amongst those who would think of themselves as your betters, self-care becomes crucial.

In chapter 10, we'll focus on accepting yourself and embracing who you are. This chapter will mainly focus on motivation and positive reinforcement. This is for every woman who feels inadequate or hopeless. We'll also look at how older women can deal with being diagnosed later in life.

In chapter 11, I will be discussing the difficulties that we as women with ADHD often face during the act of decision-making. And when we do make those choices, we often change our minds or regret the choices we've made. As you might have guessed, this causes many negative feelings that can be avoided. We'll talk about weighing pros and cons along with a collection of other tips for decision-making. We'll also discuss impulsivity in a little more detail, and tips for how to avoid impulsive decision-making will be included.

Chapter 12 will be about managing your finances. With our minds all over the place, it can be helpful to have a few tips in this regard. While a lot of other things are chaotic in our lives, our finances don't have to be.

Chapter 13 will offer practical advice on how you can manage social gatherings and food! This is not just a "woman" thing. Everyone enjoys the company of their friends and family…Okay, probably not everyone. But for those who do, formal or informal gatherings can be a storm of emotions and thoughts, to-do lists, and cooking! There will also be a few guides on how to prepare to create meals and how to make shopping for groceries easier. With a few simple steps to prepare amazing dishes, I'll also be adding a few easy recipes that can give you ideas for your next dinner party, or for when you want to cook at home. Big family, small family, married or single, everyone's gotta eat!

Let's get on with this exciting journey!

Chapter 1:

Introduction to ADHD

Attention deficit hyperactivity disorder (ADHD) is a brain disorder that affects how you pay attention, sit still, and control your behavior. It happens in children and teens and can continue into adulthood. ADHD is the most commonly diagnosed mental disorder in children. Boys are more likely to have it than girls. It's usually spotted during the early school years when a child begins to have problems paying attention.

ADHD can't be prevented or cured. But spotting it early, plus having a good treatment and education plan, can help a child or adult with ADHD manage their symptoms. This is a more compulsive behavior in adults, specifically women. These symptoms often interfere with development and functioning (Williamson, 2021).

The most common belief is that there are only three types of ADHD. However, Dr. Daniel G. Amen disagrees. Let's look at the three types that are most commonly discussed and then look at the argument that Dr. Amen states.

Types of ADHD

According to an article by Erica Roth and Kerry Weiss published on the Healthline website in October 2021, there are three most common types of ADHD. These are described as the inattentive type, the hyperactive/impulsive type, and the combination type.

The behaviors associated with ADHD can present themselves in different ways.

- **Inattention**: Very easily distracted, their concentration skills are normally lacking and they have trouble with general organization.

- **Hyperactive**: Is always fidgeting and they tend to speak faster than other people around them. They also have trouble with staying on task (Roth & Weiss, 2013).

- **Impulsivity**: Frequently interrupting others, acting without enough thought (taking a lot of risks).

With such a wide variety of people and personalities, people may experience these symptoms in different ways.

The Inattentive Type

This type of ADHD mainly struggles with inattention. While you might battle with episodes of hyperactivity or impulse control at times, these are not the main symptoms and they can normally be managed to a degree.

People who are diagnosed with this type of ADHD mainly have issues with the following:

- Easily being distracted, they might miss crucial details.

- New things might bore them after a short period of time.

- They might have trouble with keeping their thoughts organized, which makes taking on new information more difficult.

- They might frequently misplace their things.

- They may seem like they aren't listening when they "zone out."

- They might also have trouble following directions.

The Hyperactive/Impulsive Type

This type can also show signs of inattentive behavior but the most common symptoms are hyperactivity and/or impulsive behavior.

Their main symptoms may include the following:

- They may fidget or have a feeling of restlessness.

- They may have trouble sitting still for long periods of time.

- They might also speak very quickly and constantly.

- They might also be described as impatient.

- Their actions could be described as out of the blue or "out of turn" (Roth & Weiss, 2013).

The Combination Type

If you are diagnosed with this type, it means that your symptoms don't fall into either of the other two categories. You might understand this as having 50% of both symptoms.

There are those who outgrow the disorder with time and medication. But for those of us who aren't that lucky, it's a lifelong battle. The good news is that we don't necessarily have to look at it as a disorder or a battle. While we might still have certain struggles that could make most situations difficult, there are certainly ways to deal with the symptoms in a way that won't make us feel as burdensome.

The sad truth is that many people describe ADHD as a burden when it really doesn't have to be. In chapter three, we'll look at some techniques and tips for dealing with ADHD as an adult woman. These tips might change your life or, at the very least, bring some relief.

Now that you're familiar with the three most commonly diagnosed types of ADHD, let's look at Dr. Amen's argument. He believes that there are, in fact, seven types of ADHD. According to him, if you can pinpoint the exact type of ADHD, you can treat it more effectively.

Dr. Daniel Amen is a well-known author and psychiatrist. Among his many qualifications, he is also a nuclear brain imaging specialist (Louw, 2019). Dr. Amen founded eight "Amen clinics" across the United States. These clinics are devoted to diagnosing and treating the seven types of ADHD in children and adults.

The most common form of diagnosis that they use is called a SPECT scan, or Single-Photon Emission Computerized Tomography (Louw, 2019). This scan focuses on how blood flows through the brain, which allows psychiatrists to target the type of ADHD that a patient has. This, in turn, leads to specific treatment, which results in more desirable results from treatment.

Dr. Amen has diagnosed thousands of people and has come to the conclusion that there are seven types of ADHD. He actually prefers the term "ADD" which is an outdated term that was replaced in the 1980s. He feels that the term "ADD" reflects the condition in a more suitable way. For the sake of modern terminology, I will continue using the term "ADHD."

Instead of simply prescribing medications, he uses a combination of medications and lifestyle changes to treat the condition. Exercise is crucial for people who are diagnosed with ADHD (more on that later).

In an article by Keith Louw that was published in November 2019, the seven types of ADHD were summed up succinctly and clearly. Let's go over the seven types of ADHD that Dr. Amen has been researching.

"The Classic Type" (1)

The symptoms of this type are basically all three previously mentioned types combined. They can include being inattentive, easily distracted, disorganized, hyperactive, restless, and impulsive (Louw, 2019). Procrastination can also be a symptom of the classic type.

Dr. Amen's findings were that people who have the classic type have reduced blood flow in the prefrontal cortex, the cerebellum, and the basal ganglia (Louw, 2019). Treatment would need to increase dopamine levels which is done by prescribing/recommending stimulant medications, stimulant supplements, exercise, Omega-3 fatty acids, and high protein diets.

"Inattentive ADHD" (2)

According to Dr. Amen, people who have this type of ADHD often get easily distracted and they might move more slowly than others. They're rarely hyperactive and they're often described as being in a constant state of daydreaming.

Women are more commonly diagnosed with this type and it often goes undiagnosed for years because this type of ADHD does not necessarily disrupt classrooms or workplaces. These patients also have low levels of dopamine and lower activity in the prefrontal cortex, which means that the treatment is similar to the treatment for type 1.

"Overfocused ADHD" (3)

This type includes Classic ADHD symptoms but they also have trouble shifting attention. Some of their other common symptoms include:

- Overwhelming negative thoughts.

- Excessive worrying about situations or things that may not require so much thought.

- Not being very flexible with their routines or emotions.

- Frequently engages in arguments or opposes authority.

Patients who are diagnosed with overfocused ADHD suffer from low levels of serotonin and dopamine. By using treatments, Dr. Amen's goal is to increase both of these neurotransmitters, which are essentially messengers of the brain (Louw, 2019).

Anxiety is another common symptom, and because of this, Dr. Amen prefers to avoid stimulant medication because it can worsen this symptom. He prefers to treat the condition with supplements first before using medications as a last resort.

The treatments for this type of ADHD can include:

- Certain supplements
- Antidepressants
- Neurofeedback

Neurofeedback, also known as electroencephalography, is a kind of therapy that is used to measure and control your brain waves and your body temperature (Brain Forest Centers, 2019). It is thought to help "retrain" specific areas of the brain that might help fight the symptoms of ADHD and other conditions.

"Temporal Lobe ADHD" (4)

In this type, Classic ADHD symptoms are also present along with a list of other symptoms that can include:

- Irritability
- Short-tempered/aggressive
- Mood instability
- Paranoia
- Learning problems
- Memory loss
- Dark/intrusive thoughts

In these patients, Dr. Amen observed inactivity in the prefrontal cortex and different irregularities in the temporal lobe. He stated that the goal of the available treatments would be to treat the overactive cells that seem to "shoot" unpredictably and to "soothe neuronal activity" (Louw, 2019).

The treatments that Dr. Amen recommends could include supplements and a keto diet that tends to be high in fat and protein. He might also recommend and prescribe "anticonvulsant" medications to stabilize the moods of the patient.

"Limbic ADHD" (5)

Patients might not be diagnosed as early or as easily with this type of ADHD for the reason that it might present itself as depression in some cases. The symptoms that accompany this diagnosis are also similar to Classic ADHD symptoms but they also include some more prominent symptoms that make it hard to distinguish from depression. Low-level sadness might be a chronic state of mind; however, this sadness is not as severe as clinical depression.

Some of the other common symptoms include:

- Low levels of energy
- low self-esteem

Feelings of unworthiness or hopelessness can also sometimes disrupt the lives of these patients. As the name suggests, the people who have this type of ADHD have an issue with their limbic sections. Overactivity is normally the culprit. They also have inactivity in the prefrontal cortex. It has been observed that the inactivity occurs both during concentration and relaxation. The possible treatments can include exercise, supplements, and/or antidepressants.

"The Ring of Fire ADHD" (6)

Dr. Amen stresses the fact that this is a much more severe case of Classic ADHD that also has a few extra symptoms such as being sensitive to light, noise, and touch. Patients who are diagnosed with this type of ADHD may also display cyclic moodiness.

People with this type of ADHD have signs of overactivity in most parts of the brain. Treatments can include supplements and certain medications.

"Anxious ADHD" (7)

Patients who are diagnosed with this type of ADHD also display Classic ADHD symptoms that are accompanied by other symptoms such as severe anxiety and other physical symptoms that can occur because of anxiety and stress. These physical symptoms have been identified as the classic symptoms that most of us know: headaches, stomach aches, and freezing up are amongst the most common.

The basal ganglia are overactive in these patients. The basal ganglia aid the process of producing dopamine. While most other types of ADHD tend to have lower levels of dopamine, this type has higher levels. Possible treatments include supplements, medications, and neurofeedback.

Now that you know about the three classic types of ADHD and the seven more specific types of ADHD, you might be able to understand your own condition a little more. Keep in mind that self-diagnosis is never a good idea. If you suspect that you might have undiagnosed ADHD, it's important to contact a professional for the proper diagnosis and treatment plan.

How Is ADHD Diagnosed in Adults?

There is no true test for ADHD that can simply spit out a diagnosis. Your doctor would need to extensively investigate and consider multiple sources of information. Adult ADHD is often more difficult to diagnose, especially when it comes to women who might have less obvious symptoms.

ADHD isn't very common in adults and even less common in women (often because it goes undiagnosed, more on this later). For this reason, there wasn't always oodles of information or help available. Luckily, that has slowly been changing in recent years. If you don't know how to get in contact with the right kind of specialist, your primary healthcare practitioner can help you with referrals and information.

Here is a list of possible methods of diagnosis:

Psychological Tests

These tests can be checklists or other tests that can also be used to determine whether you might have any kind of other disabilities that could be mistaken for ADHD. You might also get checked out for anxiety and depression, which can occur along with ADHD.

Detailed Questions

The doctor could possibly ask numerous questions relating to symptoms and how they affect your daily life and functioning. These questions will likely revolve around your workplace and relationships, among other things. During this session, it's important to answer all the questions as honestly as you can. Try not to let guilt or shame stand in the way of your diagnosis. Your doctor can't give you the support you need if he does not know all the details.

Keep in mind that the more details you offer, the higher the chances are that they may be able to diagnose you with the correct type of ADHD as well. A Dr. Amen stated, knowing which type of ADHD you have will definitely aid in knowing the type of treatment you need.

Looking at Past Events

In order for your doctor to fully understand the scale of the situation, they might need to question you about your childhood as well. ADHD generally starts in early childhood, even if symptoms might have been different at the time. In women, symptoms might not have become apparent enough to notice until well into adulthood. Since ADHD starts during childhood, experts agree that adults are not likely to develop the condition at random.

Along with these methods and the non-invasive "SPECT" that I discussed earlier, the doctor might also request speaking to important people in your life who are close to you and might therefore have observed certain behavior. Rest assured, this is in your best interest and you shouldn't feel embarrassed or ashamed.

What Causes ADHD?

Even in this modern time that we live in, the exact causes of ADHD are still not known. There are a few factors that can play a role and seem to be linked to the condition. Genetics is thought to be the most easily explainable possible cause. We understand that many mental health conditions may be inherited from family members, especially parents. Addiction, depression, anxiety, and other conditions are among those that can be classified as gene-related.

For this reason, it's clearly an easy assumption to make when it comes to ADHD. What started out as an assumption might have become more evidence-based over the years as family members with the same condition were traced. If you have a family history of ADHD, it might be in your best interest to reach out to a professional sooner rather than later.

According to Dr. Amen's work, it can also be assumed that the differences in brain activity could also be a possible cause. There is some speculation about whether babies who were born prematurely might be at a higher risk than the average person. This debate has not been settled.

There is also some advice that suggests that the risk of developing ADHD might be heightened by prenatal exposures such as alcohol and tobacco (American Academy of Pediatrics, 2019). The same source states that head injuries or even toxins such as lead could also be to blame.

Are You a Worried Mother or Family Member?

You likely decided to conduct research on this topic because of your own condition. Now that you have a clearer understanding, you might be wondering about your children or the children of family members. Since I discussed genetics as playing a possible role in causing ADHD, it's natural for you to wonder about it.

Rest assured that none of the above-mentioned possibilities have been 100% verified. Even if you do notice symptoms in these children, you now know that there are many different treatment options available. Too many parents feel like failures because of their children's essentially unavoidable conditions. This condition is not a life sentence, and a good quality of life is more than possible.

You also understand the symptoms and you know what to look out for now. Symptoms in children are very similar to those in adults. Affected children might be disruptive and they might even seem difficult to handle. All that they need is a proper diagnosis, treatment, and patience.

Patience is one of the most important keys to successfully raising a child with ADHD. Regardless of how difficult to manage these children might seem, you need to remember that no child is a bad child. You'll be surprised at how much of a difference the right treatment can make.

People sometimes overlook girls with symptoms of ADHD because they might not be as disruptive as the boys. However, that's not the case for all girls. Some of them can be just as hyperactive as the boys. Girls tend to handle or mask their symptoms better than boys do.

For this reason, it's important to pay an equal amount of attention to all children who display symptoms, even if the symptoms seem insignificant at the time. Girls who go undiagnosed might struggle with a lack of coping mechanisms until well into adulthood. As their responsibilities increase and the pressure mounts, they might find it more difficult to stay on top of every situation. Again, diagnosis and treatment are key!

Offering support to a diagnosed child or family member is just as crucial. People/children who have this condition may feel overwhelmed in many situations, as you well know. Offering love and guidance is a sure way to help relieve the feeling. As a parent or family member, you need to remember that listening to how a child feels is a great way to offer support. When you think about your own battles and what you wish more people did for you, these are the things that you can do for other people with the same condition.

Under-diagnosed and under-treated girls with ADHD face distinct risks.

Depression, anxiety, failing at school or college, self-harm, unemployment, unplanned pregnancies, and an even greater chance of dying young.

The dangers and devastating impact of suffering associated with attention-deficit/hyperactivity disorder, or ADHD, are enormous. It costs billions of dollars in missed productivity and healthcare spending each year, as well as unfathomable despair and failure.

Despite more than a century of study and dozens of published studies, the public still has a poor understanding of ADHD, which is characterized by inattention, forgetfulness, and impulsivity. This is true, especially for females and girls.

Pediatricians, schools, and parents have grown much better at detecting ADHD in females over the last several decades. Scientists believed it was up to nine times more frequent in boys in the 1990s, and relatively few girls were identified. Today's diagnostic rate is 2.5 males for every 1 female.

Even still, an ongoing issue lingers. Whilst most males with ADHD tend to be more physically active and impulsive, features physicians refer to as "hyperactive," many girls with the disease tend to be more introverted, dreamyr, and distracted—or, in clinical lingo, "inattentive." Experts believe that many females with ADHD are still being unnoticed—and hence going untreated—in part because of these milder symptoms.

"Who gets detected as having ADHD?" wonders Stephen Hinshaw, a psychologist at the University of California, Berkeley who is a major researcher on ADHD in females. "You're referred to if you're conspicuous, if you're interfering with others." Boys are more likely than females to have aggressiveness and impulsive issues. As a result, girls who have inattentive difficulties are not regarded to have ADHD." Instead, he claims, educators and others think the issue is worry or family problems.

Hinshaw began researching females with ADHD in 1997 as part of a federally financed project known as the Berkeley Girls with ADHD Longitudinal Study (B-GALS). As he and his colleagues tracked their participants into adulthood, they discovered that females with ADHD had most of the same issues as males with the condition, as well as some additional things.

One of the unique burdens of girls is evading notice. Women and girls, in general, participate in more "internalizing" behavior than males, according to Hinshaw, which means they prefer to blame themselves rather than others for their issues. Girls with ADHD experience higher anxiety and sadness than males with the disease or girls without it.

Another important longitudinal research on females, performed by Harvard physician and scientist Joseph Biederman, discovered that serious depression is more than twice as likely in teen girls with ADHD than in girls without the disease.

According to the research, girls with ADHD are considerably more likely than boys with ADHD or other females to self-harm, including slashing and burning themselves, and to contemplate suicide. Furthermore, while teenage boys with ADHD are more prone than girls with the disease to consume illicit substances, women with the disorder are more likely to become engaged in violent relationships.

Another significant issue for females with ADHD is hazardous sexual conduct, which leads to alarmingly high rates of unintended births. According to research, more than 40% of young women have ADHD, compared to 10% of young women who do not have ADHD. Hinshaw and UC Berkeley psychologist Elizabeth Owens connected unplanned births to worse academic attainment early in life in the most recent B-GALS update, released in 2019.

"Daily, girls and women blame themselves more," says Ellen Littman, a clinical psychologist in Mount Kisco, New York, who publishes and lectures regularly on girls and women with ADHD. "If a male fails an exam, he may comment, 'What a ridiculous test,' but a lady may reply, 'I'm an idiot.' Girls are frequently quite skilled at masking their feelings of being different, bewildered, and overwhelmed."

Attention Control

Attention deficit hyperactivity disorder (ADHD) is estimated to affect more than 6 million children and 10 million adults in the United States. Most people with the illness have normal intellect; although ADHD has been linked to slightly lower IQ scores, Hinshaw believes this is due to how IQ is measured. Some people with ADHD have high IQs, he claims.

Several women with ADHD report being able to focus intensively when they are interested, and they appreciate their inventiveness. (According to Hinshaw, the data on creativity is equivocal, leaving unanswered the question of whether ADHD helps people think creatively outside the box or if persons with the disease are often too chaotic to benefit from their uncommon ideas.)

Some doctors, like Hinshaw, believe the term ADHD is misleading. He regards the disease as more of a difficulty managing attention, particularly in changing contexts, than as a weakness in and of itself.

The dark side, on the other hand, is undeniably present for both females and boys. Russell A. Barkley and Mariellen Fischer conducted recent research in which they compared 131 young individuals with ADHD to 71 control cases, to use a life insurance actuarial model to predict life expectancy. According to the findings, which were published in the *Journal of Attention* in July 2019, individuals with the most severe condition of ADHD may have their life expectancy decreased by up to 12.7 years. Barkley, a child psychologist and researcher at Virginia Commonwealth University Medical Center, explains the conclusion by citing studies that demonstrate students with ADHD are less attentive and diligent, more likely to follow poor eating habits and be overweight, and much more likely to commit suicide. Other investigations have discovered an increased risk of premature mortality.

Aside from the numerous misconceptions surrounding women with ADHD, another widely held belief is that ADHD is only found in youngsters. According to Hinshaw, Barkley, and other studies, at least half of people diagnosed as children still exhibit ADHD symptoms as adults. Indeed, Hinshaw discovered that in recent years, women have sought diagnoses in virtually similar numbers as males, frequently after noticing symptoms of the strongest genetic condition in their children.

While keeping an eye on these changes, Hinshaw and other researchers have urged parents and teachers to improve their ability to recognize girls who are suffering and to design treatments that improve academic achievement, boost self-esteem, and help women avoid dangerous behaviors.

There's an Issue in the Classroom

Despite the belief that ADHD is a late-twentieth-century issue, the Scottish physician Albert Crichton reported an "unnatural or pathological sensitivity of the nerves" generating exceptional distraction more than two centuries ago. Crichton hypothesized in 1798 that what he labeled "the illness of attention" may be caused by inheritance or accident.

Hinshaw observes that as compulsory schooling extended across Europe and the United States, children who struggled to focus in an institutional environment were more at a disadvantage.

According to Hinshaw, the growth of public institutions meant that "every youngster had to attend class." "And do you know what? A strikingly constant proportion of children in Europe and the United States struggle with focusing, sitting still, and learning to read."

Having early childhood education now mandated in many parts of the world, the estimated incidence of ADHD in most nations varies from 5 to 7 percent, according to Hinshaw. The rates of diagnosis differ very substantially. The United States has one of the highest rates in the world, with one in every nine children being diagnosed, and it is a major source of contention.

The condition has gone under several names over the years, notably "hyperkinetic impulse disorder" and "minimal brain malfunction." It wasn't until 1980 that "attention deficit disorder" (ADD), the first label to emphasize distraction, was included in the Diagnostic and Statistical Manual of Mental Disorders (DSM), the handbook relied upon by mental health practitioners worldwide. A second DSM edition altered the label to "attention-deficit/hyperactivity disorder," or ADHD, seven years later.

ADHD is a spectrum condition that includes both persons with minor deficiencies and those with severe impairments. Researchers currently categorize people as hyper, forgetful, or a mix of the two. Men are much more likely to be classified as hyperactive, whereas women are more likely to be classified as distracted or a mix of sluggish and overactive.

According to a 2018 British research that compared parents' views with more objective data, the signs of inattentive females may be easier to notice, but observers' biases may also contribute to under-diagnosis. The study, which included 283 diagnosed males and females, discovered that parents view ADHD-related traits significantly in males and females, underrating hyperactivity and impulsivity in females while magnifying such features in males. "The diagnostic criteria [are] based on masculine behaviors," explains Florence Mowlem, a health consultant who researched as part of her doctoral studies at King's College in London. "Perhaps we need something different for ladies."

After carefully analyzing applicants with questions and eight-hour evaluation sessions, Hinshaw and colleagues chose 140 girls aged 6 to 12 years old with both inattentive and mixed ADHD, as well as 88 girls without the disease. For three years, the girls joined a five-week camp that included art and acting lessons as well as outdoor activities.

Throughout this time, the diagnosed females volunteered to forego medicine.

The researchers watched the women's interactions and assessed their IQs, anxiety levels, and interpersonal skills. Their first paper, published in the *Journal of Consulting and Clinical Psychology* in 2002, showed how females with the condition struggled to control their thoughts, feelings, and actions. They also had the same types of academic difficulties as males with the illness. According to Hinshaw, in other fields such as arithmetic, girls performed significantly worse than their male counterparts.

The girls' social life was also harmed. Researchers discovered that girls with a mixed presentation of ADHD were frequently hated and rejected by their friends, which Hinshaw describes as "devastating." According to him, such social isolation can cause females to lose self-esteem and raise their chances of participating in antisocial conduct, such as substance abuse.

When Hinshaw's team watched the girls as teens years later, they discovered that the majority of the girls' childhood deficits had persisted. During this period, just a few of the females improved in math, memory, or planning. Furthermore, several new issues have surfaced, such as eating problems, attempted suicide, and self-harm, which Hinshaw associates with ADHD-related impulsivity.

Unsolved Conundrums

Patricia Quinn, a former developmental pediatrician who previously worked at Georgetown University Medical Center in Washington, DC, has written extensively about ADHD in women and girls. She has worked with dozens of adult women who suffered from disorganization, poor planning, social issues, and distraction without recognizing that it was due to ADHD. "I believe there is still a lot of misconception and misdiagnosis concerning the condition," she says. Quinn, who has been diagnosed with ADHD, believes that such news "may be an encouraging diagnosis. These ladies can be helped and have extremely prosperous lives."

It is undeniable that ADHD medicine benefits a large number of people. However, "It's seldom an acceptable long-term answer on its own," adds Hinshaw. "Even if it is effective, it is not a solution." Learning communication skills, for example, is a critical component of conquering the illness. In adults, positive data indicate that cognitive behavioral treatment improves organizational and time management abilities, as well as mood control.

Hinshaw's B-GALS study was funded for 23 years by the National Institute of Mental Health, but Hinshaw claims the project is currently on hold until his staff can seek a suitable backer. His ambition is to conduct a fifth follow-up study on the females, who are in their thirties. According to the UC Berkeley team and other academics in the subject, there are still many mysteries to be solved. As an example: Why do men and women experience ADHD in different ways? What causes it to be somewhat severe? Which brain structures or hormones are more important? Is there a more objective technique to diagnose ADHD and assess the efficacy of various treatments? Most importantly, how else can our health and education institutions do a superior job of relieving pain and stigma for both men and women?

Some progress has been made. According to research, there is indeed a significant genetic component; however, exactly also how many genes are involved is unknown, and it is evident that environment also has a role. Gender variations in neurobiology may also help clarify some of the discrepancies in how males and females experience ADHD. Researchers compared the brains of ADHD men and women to their neurotypical counterparts three years earlier. The volume and form of the globus pallidus and the amygdala, two brain areas critical for emotions, were shown to be altered in males with ADHD but not in women.

Hormonal variations may also be a factor. "Estrogen levels appear to influence ADHD symptomatology in women," Quinn explains. However, she observes that there are more problems than solutions at this stage.

The way ahead, according to Hinshaw, is to teach teachers, parents, physicians, and especially youngsters with ADHD how to spot it and its symptoms in both women and men. "We might be able to have a completely different set of ideas about mental health and developmental disorders in a generation or two as those kids grow up to be adults," he adds.

Chapter 2:

How ADHD Presents in Women

Let's dive deeper into why women can sometimes go undiagnosed for years. As mentioned before, women often have fewer disruptive symptoms. Even when they do have symptoms that are quite obvious, these symptoms tend to be labeled as personality traits, or they might even be misdiagnosed as other conditions.

While it's true that other mental health disorders can coexist along with ADHD, it still needs to be individually diagnosed (more on this later). Other symptoms can make this difficult, especially in women. Women also tend to be less aggressive, whereas men can have issues with that aspect.

Chances are that if you're reading this, you chose a book specifically written for women because you've noticed the gender gap.

Differences in Men and Women

Women deserve to be heard when they cry out for help but are instead dismissed. A lot of women don't even understand what they're going through. With so many people telling you that you're "fine" or that it's just a little anxiety, some women may begin to feel as though there might be something wrong with them. Let me tell you, having ADHD does not mean that there is something wrong with you.

It simply means that your brain is different. If women don't understand ADHD and what kinds of symptoms it can present, they might spend their lives trying to cope under immense amounts of stress and pressure. There is so much pressure on women to be calm and collected. Women have to be the "good cops." This is, as mentioned before, a major reason for misdiagnosis. Women who go undiagnosed can further suffer from immense inner conflict. Since some of the symptoms that women experience can be mistaken for personality traits, they might also begin to believe this false accusation.

This leads to bottled-up emotions that can often trigger outbursts at home, away from the eyes of society. These outbursts, in turn, lead to further demotivation and low self-esteem.

Women also tend to feel as though they don't need a support system because they often take the role of the support system. When you're always putting the needs of others above your own, you need to ask yourself who will be looking after your own needs.

Because of these social standards, some women might suppress or mask their symptoms until much later in life when they've become nearly unbearable. Now, if you've researched the topic before, you've probably read that ADHD presents itself similarly in men and women.

Most articles or books explain that the number of symptoms and the severity of symptoms are mostly the same for both sexes. From personal experience, that's just not true. If you're here because you've been diagnosed, then you will probably agree. If you're here but you are yet to be diagnosed, then it's a new fact that you'll learn today.

While it's always good to mention that this does not include every single woman, it does make up the majority of the group. Another reason for women going undiagnosed or being misdiagnosed might be a reluctance to reach out for the necessary help. When you've been told over and over again that a feeling is simply anxiety, your mind might start wandering and you might feel as though shutting others out might be your only option. For this reason, I want to implore you once again to reach out to professionals if you feel that there might be something more to blame.

Women with ADHD are often intelligent perfectionists. During childhood, they might have achieved many academic awards or other related accomplishments. As they get older and the symptoms change, making concentration more difficult, it takes a lot more effort and time to achieve the same kinds of high standards.

When further demotivation kicks in, these women can then start questioning whether they really do have the abilities in which they pride themselves. They might feel as though they are less capable because the people around them seem to function much faster and easier than they do.

Firstly, that's utter nonsense. You are more than capable of anything that you set your mind to. Recognizing that you might have ADHD is the first step, but the important step is realizing that it doesn't matter how long it takes you to complete a task. What matters is the impeccable quality, which you are capable of delivering.

By keeping your internal struggles to yourself, you're essentially robbing yourself. With so many women hellbent on appearing as if they have their s#*t together all the time, it can be tempting to want to follow suit. Remember, just because your symptoms are less obvious, that doesn't make them less damaging if left untreated.

Let's look at some common differences between symptoms in men and women.

Self-efficacy: Since we now know that women and girls who have ADHD tend to have problems with their self-esteem, we can assume that this puts them at a higher risk of depression. The concept of "self-efficacy" was first used by Albert Bandura who was a professor in psychology at Stanford University. It refers to someone's belief in their own ability to execute the necessary behaviors to produce specific performance attainments (Carey & Forsyth, 2009).

In simpler terms, it refers to the belief in your ability to control your own motivation, social environment, and behavior (Carey & Forsyth, 2009). In most of my research, I've found that women with ADHD are said to have lower self-efficacy than men. As one can imagine, this can make life incredibly difficult for the women who experience the symptom.

Not only does it cause inner turmoil, but it can also cause physical issues that could have been avoided with the proper treatment and support. Chances are, you've probably felt this way over your lifetime. It's normal but unfortunate. Most of the women who experience this symptom don't realize their true potential.

Men tend to have fewer struggles with the more emotional side of ADHD (not none, just fewer). While men do suffer from mental health disorders and their feelings and problems are still valid, the truth is that it affects women on a deeper level, in this case.

Coping strategies: My research has also led me to believe that women and girls tend to have fewer coping strategies than boys or men. This does not make us any less capable; the fact that we have fewer coping strategies only further proves that women are too easily overlooked in this situation. The proper strategies and techniques can be learned if these women have access to the help that they need.

Now, this next difference is a fact that I came across that stunned me for a moment. According to some researchers, men with ADHD are more often incarcerated than women with ADHD (Carey & Forsyth, 2009).

I wouldn't really call it a fact, perhaps more of an observation. Since men who have ADHD tend to be more aggressive and disruptive (as you now know), I can see how this might have come to light. In reality, the studies that have been conducted on gender differences can't all be taken as 100% factual, as the studies were often of small groups instead of a large enough sample of people.

One can assume that the only way to truly understand the differences would be to experience them yourself.

Verbal aggression: There is some evidence that suggests that women and girls who have ADHD can sometimes be more verbally aggressive (Kinman, 2016). This is more common in adolescence since most of us (hopefully) outgrow the verbal-bully mindset as we grow older. What this teaches us is that if you notice a child who tends to be a bit of a verbal bully, you should understand that it's likely a call for help from a child who does not understand how to control their emotions.

Treatment: This is not a symptom but simply an observation about treatment referral. We know that women often don't get the proper diagnosis or that they might not reach out for help. But judging from my research, even women who do get diagnosed are very likely to not get referred for proper treatment.

What makes this difficult for these women is the fact that they know that they have a logical explanation for their struggles, yet they don't seem to have a big enough problem to receive any kind of help. Feelings of unworthiness might result from this, or they might not fully grasp the extent of their condition, which in turn will lead to further suffering without relief.

Again, it all comes down to how the patient presents symptoms. Symptoms also are not enough to make a proper diagnosis. In all honesty, there is a great shortage of studies that review the differences between men and women who have ADHD. In my opinion, much further research would be necessary to fully understand how all the differences play a role.

If professionals in the area took more time to properly research the topic, we might have more extensive and personalized treatments. While there are doctors and psychologists who dedicate their lives to truly helping men and women who live with this condition and to researching new ways of doing that, they're few in numbers when compared to the professionals who stick to what they know.

Let's Talk About Comorbid Conditions

As you now know, anxiety is a common misdiagnosis in women with ADHD. Here's the thing: it can also be a comorbid condition. Some women can have one or more conditions that further mask the symptoms of ADHD.

Here are some of the most common comorbid conditions:

- Depression
- Anxiety disorders
- Bipolar disorder
- Substance use disorder
- Personality disorders

These conditions are common along with ADHD, and they make it more difficult to diagnose ADHD because of their symptoms that seem to be overlapping. The most common comorbid condition is bipolar disorder. "Rates of ADHD comorbidity in bipolar disorder have been estimated between 9.5% and 21.2%, and rates of comorbid bipolar disorder in ADHD at 5.1% and 47.1%" (Katzman et al., 2017).

Another interesting fact is that 18% of adults who are diagnosed with both ADHD and depression and 23% of adults who are diagnosed with ADHD and bipolar disorder are roughly calculated to also have a kind of personality disorder (Katzman et al., 2017).

Okay, you might be starting to feel a little worried here. Firstly, there is no reason to be worried. Your mental health matters, and it should be important to you and your loved ones. Being diagnosed with more than one condition, again, does not mean that there is something wrong with you. Mental health disorders should not be something to be ashamed of or afraid of.

Being diagnosed also doesn't mean that you are any less capable of living an extraordinary life or climbing to amazing heights. As long as you get the help that you need, you have nothing to worry about.

There are common misconceptions about doctors and medications that need to be put down. There isn't anything shameful about having to take certain medications. And the doctors who prescribe them do so in order to help you be the best version of yourself.

Some people argue that medications for mental health disorders are all part of some money-making scam. From personal experience, this is not the case. Your doctor is highly qualified in their field, and if they suggest medications or other forms of treatments, it would be wiser to take their advice in higher regard than the advice of the Karen next door.

Truthfully, in some cases, there are treatment options that might offer more benefits than medications. If you're still uncomfortable with medication, you can always raise your concerns and ask for more information. Being more informed on your options might aid in your own peace of mind.

Experiences of Real Women: A Bit of Advice

As a woman who has been diagnosed with ADHD myself, I have been a part of support groups on Facebook for a long time. During this time, I have read many stories and struggles of women all over the world. Their stories have helped me feel less alone, and being able to relate to them so much has really made a difference.

I want to suggest joining support groups on social media for this reason. Being an adult woman with ADHD can feel like an incredibly lonely journey. I assure you, you are not alone! It's from these support groups that I have also come to understand a great deal about how ADHD can present itself in adult women.

I want to share some of the struggles that I have read about. Respecting the privacy of these women, unfortunately, means that I won't be using any names or the names of the specific support groups.

One of the most common issues that women from all around the world seem to deal with would be heightened emotions. I have read testimonies upon testimonies of women who understand that their feelings might be out of proportion. These women understand that the given situations might not be as intense as they initially feel them to be, but they explain that their emotions regarding the situations can sometimes still be overwhelming.

One such post that I came across was about a young woman who expressed her annoyance with her partner who refused to attend a social gathering that would require him to dress formally. She explained that she knew that it was essentially his decision to accompany her or not, but that the frustration she felt at that moment was difficult to cope with.

To most women, such a situation would invoke negative emotions to a point, but the way she explained her anger and frustration would be difficult to understand for someone who doesn't fully grasp the scale of how much deeper we feel things.

If you've noticed a similar kind of feeling, don't be alarmed. It's a perfectly normal symptom that can be treated and dealt with, often by learning helpful calming techniques (more on this later).

Another benefit of these support groups is that these women often bring a little humor into their posts. It can feel like a dreary situation if you only focus on the negative. I have to admit that it is quite refreshing to read about stories relating to symptoms such as forgetfulness.

Forgetfulness is another one of the most common symptoms in adult women. I had to swallow the urge to giggle out loud on the bus from reading about another young woman who often lost her underwear. She expressed her frustration in such a humorous way that made it both relatable and entertaining.

Unfortunately, along with all the interesting and relatable stories of daydreaming and "zoning out," there are also posts about the darker side of ADHD in women. From what I have read, women who have ADHD can often have a lot of anger built up inside of them. This also relates to having heightened emotions but on an even greater scale.

This kind of built-up anger can lead to unhealthy coping mechanisms such as self-harm or substance abuse, especially when ADHD is paired with other comorbid conditions. In your quest to deal with your ADHD, it's important to remember that it's okay to not always understand your emotions or to not always have the answers. That's why we have our doctors who can, over time, become our very anchor to reality.

Another common symptom in women is having trouble with impulsive shopping. We're probably all more guilty of this than we'd like to admit. While spoiling yourself or loved ones now and then is perfectly normal and good, you need to sit down and work out a budget for yourself to keep you on track (she said while knowing full well that she went way over budget with buying new clothes for her kids the previous day). *Okay*, so nobody is perfect!

With that being said, you should never beat yourself up for any kind of slip-up. In the end, you're still a human being, and in the words of my dear friend Grammarly, "To err is to human." Your goal should be to improve yourself as much as you can, but not even your average Joe with no traces of ADHD or any other kind of mental condition never has a setback.

Your setbacks shouldn't weigh you down because they don't define your progress. That's another reason why these support groups have been so helpful. Women from all over who have similar struggles or different struggles build each other up and support one another regardless of whether they're complete strangers or not.

It's inspiring to read about so many women who have fallen and stood right back up again. Sharing your own experiences in a safe space with like-minded people also lifts an enormous burden from your shoulders. Even if you join purely to read about other people and their journeys without wanting to share your own, that's okay, too. It's still worth a shot!

For the purpose of research and insight, I decided to create a list of questions that I planned on presenting to the two support groups of which I am a member. I wanted to pose the questions to real women in order to get the type of answers that you can't exactly find with other forms of research.

While we are exploring some of these questions in detail throughout this book, I want to hear what women have to say when given the option to anonymously give their opinions and experiences.

Here are the questions:

1. Have you been diagnosed?

2. What symptoms led you to suspect ADHD?

3. How old were you when you were diagnosed?

4. Were you ever misdiagnosed?

5. Who diagnosed you? (doctor, etc.)

6. How were you diagnosed? (What did the doctor ask or do to diagnose you?)

7. What treatments were available to you? (Medication or others, and which type of medications)

8. Did you have any side effects from treatments?

9. Did you ever feel as if you were being overlooked because of your gender (women are frequently misdiagnosed or overlooked because symptoms can manifest differently than in men)

10. Do you have any comorbid conditions?

11. Do you have trouble with romantic relationships, work, or your social life?

12. How do you cope as a mother with ADHD? (if you have children; fur babies count!)

13. Do you think your life would have been different if you did not have the condition?

14. Has the condition held you back from achieving your goals?

15. What would you say your greatest weakness is?

16. What would you say your biggest strength is?

17. Tell us a funny story about your life with ADHD!

The Answers

I'm going to be placing their individual answers below for you to read through. This might add a bit of entertainment to your day (provided funny stories) or help you understand how other women feel.

Anonymous A

1. "Yes"

2. "I'm not sure, my mom says I was very hyper. Apparently, I gave the boys a run for their money."

3. "I was small, I think 7 or 8."

4. "No, ADHD was the first thing that the doctor suspected."

5. "I'm not too sure, he was a doctor."

6. "I can't really remember, he spoke to me and my mom and asked a bunch of questions."

7. "I was put on medication, Concerta."

8. "Not that I can remember, and not now, either."

9. "When I was younger, I didn't really notice anything. I was just a kid. It was normal for me. I grew up with ADHD. When I got older I started having problems that I felt were because of ADHD. My doctor didn't seem to take me seriously; it felt like it, anyway."

10. "I was diagnosed with depression when I was 22."

11. "Yes, work has been hard. I struggle with keeping on top of my work and I have a short temper. My relationships were all pretty negative, too."

12. "I don't have kids. I can't imagine having to take care of them and myself right now. I have a pet snake, he keeps to himself."

13. "Maybe, I feel pretty normal. Probably because I don't know anything else. But I do blame ADHD for my last relationship failing. That's why I saw the doctor."

14. "I can't concentrate for very long, and I procrastinate a lot."

15. "Hey, I can make a mean pasta dish. That probably doesn't have anything to do with ADHD."

16. "Oh! Don't get me started, I have so many. When I was 17 I stood in line at a food court to get hotdogs with my best friend. The line was long and I got distracted so once I got to the counter, my friend ordered our hotdogs and I swayed along with her, my thoughts were super lost in space. When she handed me my hotdog I was not paying attention and well… I stuck my hand out (it was like an autopilot movement) and dropped the thing. I mean, it probably doesn't sound all that funny now. But at that moment, the chaos of me scrambling to catch it and my friend jumping to get away, well, it was kind of funny."

Anonymous B

1. "Yes"

2. "When I was a kid, I always seemed to be more hyper than the rest of the kids. I would frequently get into trouble by my kindergarten teachers for being unable to take naps with the rest."

3. "I was diagnosed at the age of 9."

4. "No, never."

5. "Our doctor we always went to when I was a kid."

6. "He asked me and my father a few questions like about how active I was, did I like to keep my hands busy and such."

7. "I was given Focalin XR."

8. "Not that I can remember, none."

9. "I felt like people didn't really care that I was diagnosed with ADHD. I was actually told once by a male friend that it's all just in my head and that I seek attention."

10. "At the age of 19 I was diagnosed with both anxiety and depression."

11. "I do, because of my anxiety I get super anxious thinking that my partner is going to leave me. It hasn't really affected my work much honestly, but definitely my social life. I struggle to keep up with conversation, I become restless and agitated."

12. "I have a Siberian husky as a pet and Leyla, my dog, actually helps me. She is very talkative and active, but I become anxious without her."

13. "I think it would've been quite different. Depression and anxiety, including my ADHD, does create this wall for me in life. I think I would've been more of an extrovert and full of life."

14. "It has set some obstacles in my way, but never prevented me from achieving any goals."

15. "My greatest weakness is definitely sitting still. I can't seem to stay still for over five minutes and it does irritate many people. I dread having to go to functions such as weddings, funerals, etc. It makes me look disrespectful."

16. "My biggest strength is definitely my determination to fight depression, anxiety, and some of my ADHD symptoms. As I mentioned before, I have a lot of determination to reach my life goals and fight off the negative feelings."

Anonymous C

1. "Yes, I have been diagnosed."

2. "Exhaustion and fidgeting as a child made my dad concerned."

3. "I was 13 when I got diagnosed."

4. "I actually was misdiagnosed with autism at the age of 10, but over 3 years we noticed my symptoms did not match autism symptoms."

5. "A doctor diagnosed me, different from the first docs who misdiagnosed me."

6. "I was asked some questions and examined. My father was asked about how active I was, which I was very slow and grumpy from mostly being tired."

7. "I was given Desoxyn to treat my ADHD."

8. "I did, yes. After a while I would randomly twitch that we actually thought something else was wrong with me."

9. "That didn't actually come to mind, but thinking about it I do think so since I was misdiagnosed for autism instead of ADHD because my symptoms were different."

10. "None no."

11. "Not really. Just trouble handling my sluggishness which makes it hard to concentrate."

12. "Since I'm still a spring chicken, I only have two cats. Mew and Tux. I don't really have a struggle caring for them."

13. "I'm not sure, it might've been, but since I don't know how it feels without ADHD completely, it's hard to say."

14. "No none. I always strive to reach my goals. Well, maybe my dream of becoming an athlete, but I'm much too tired for it."

15. "My insecurity about being seen as lazy due to my tiredness."

16. "I don't think I have one at all. There isn't really something that stands out to me."

Anonymous D

1. "I am, yes."

2. "I always thought I was just quiet and liked to be creative with my hands, but my parents became worried when I became older. Especially that I always kept playing with the zipper of my jackets or anything to keep my hands busy with."

3. "I was only diagnosed at the age of 15 since I was misdiagnosed twice."

4. "Unfortunately, I have been misdiagnosed twice."

5. "Coincidentally, the same doctor who misdiagnosed me twice."

6. "The doctor did a more thorough examination of me like questions, checked my social life, and how active I was."

7. "I was prescribed Dexedrine."

8. "Definitely the loss of appetite."

9. "Yes, definitely. Because I was misdiagnosed twice, I feel like women are just pushed aside. It makes me a bit upset, because I was diagnosed only at the age of 15. Mostly because ADHD has caused some trouble for me and now that it's in control, many teens tell me I was just seeking attention."

10. "Depression is definitely in the air."

11. "Romantically, I don't think it will work for me. When I was on a date at the age of 18, I forgot to take my medication to help with my fidgeting. I was too excited. While we were eating out I started to get fidgety. The place we went to had these buttons you press when you want to call the waiter. Me being fidgety, I took the button and started pressing it repeatedly. My date didn't see what I was doing as I didn't want to let him know. Soon enough a very angry manager came and asked if we read the rules. My date looked confused and asked what was going on. The manager said we keep pressing the button which is starting to irritate and stress out the staff. I immediately stopped pressing the button and gently placed it on the floor so they wouldn't notice it. I nervously laughed and looked around on the table saying that it must've fallen off the table and got stuck causing rapid button pressing. That was the last time I went on a date. For now. Maybe."

12. "Don't have a pet or children."

13. "I don't know honestly. I still got treated the same when I was misdiagnosed and after I was diagnosed."

14. "Definitely from having friends."

15. "Being able to stop fidgeting at important times."

16. "I honestly feel that I don't have any, but if I'd look deeply it's most likely my endurance and acceptance of how I'm treated."

Anonymous E

1. "Yes."

2. "I struggle to pay attention."

3. "I was diagnosed at the age of 6."

4. "Luckily I've never been misdiagnosed."

5. "A doctor."

6. "Since I struggled to even pay attention to the doctor for the questions, it was one of the giveaways."

7. "Can't remember the name, but it was to keep focussed."

8. "Not from what I can remember, no."

9. "I do feel many women get overlooked for ADHD, but I was lucky enough to have a doctor that saw it fast."

10. "Depression and anxiety."

11. "I have trouble focusing all the time at work."

12. "Don't have a fur baby or children."

13. "A hard question to answer, but probably yes."

14. "No never."

15. "Lack of paying attention."

16. "Being able to control most of my ADHD."

I've listened to other fellow women with ADHD and they make me feel confident. It is interesting to see how different yet similar it is for women. Let this inspire and empower you as a woman! We are all sisters in arms!

Chapter 3:

Tips and Techniques to Help Women Deal With ADHD

Now that you know some of the common facts about ADHD and the struggles that women face, we can start discussing some ways that can help fight these issues. The first two chapters introduced you to the basics so that you can understand that what you're dealing with is normal and nothing to be ashamed of.

Planning

Any situation that you wish to overcome requires planning. The easiest way to navigate through some of the things that might make life harder for you would be to plan out simple steps to help guide you in the right direction. Planning to properly manage your time, ways to avoid procrastination, and ways to regulate your emotions are all good places to start.

Time Management

You might not know it, but getting enough hours of shut-eye is the first step to proper time management. You're less likely to fall behind on your schedule if you've had enough rest.

You might have heard that keeping a diary is a good way to help you with your time management. You might have thought that it was a creative and helpful idea, or you might have thought that it's a total waste of time.

In my experience, it really does work. Not only will writing down your appointments and duties for the day help you manage your time, but it'll also help you to not forget the important things! We all struggle with forgetfulness. If you can write down your responsibilities for the day in your diary, along with other seemingly insignificant things, you're more likely to remember them. Even if you do forget, regularly checking your diary will still refresh your memory.

Another way of managing your time is to create a routine that works for you and stick to it! Routines become second nature after a while. Think about your morning routine, you might wake up and have a cup of coffee before your shower. Never a shower before your coffee. That's a routine that's become embedded into your subconscious. It's not like you planned these things, they kind of just happened. Creating a new routine that allows you enough time spent on certain activities or projects should help you stay on track with your time.

You can customize and chop and change your routine(s) as much as you'd like until they suit your individual needs and daily schedule.

Here's an example of my routine when I'm working from home.

I wake up at 6:30 a.m., have a cup of coffee, and then brush my teeth. I go to the gym for 40 minutes and then have a shower at home before having my breakfast. This is the same morning routine I follow every day.

After my morning routine, my work routine begins. I focus on work from 9:00 a.m. to about 11:00 a.m. and then grant myself a half-hour break. After my break, I focus on work for another two hours, followed by another half-hour break. This is how I spend most of my days.

I also break up my work into smaller sections. I might spend two hours on research and the next two hours might be spent on writing. Now, women who don't work from home might have a different kind of routine. Whatever works for you is the right way to go. As long as you create a functional routine and commit to it.

I also tend to set about a hundred reminders for myself on my cell phone. Not just so that I know when it's time to take a break or to start working again but to remind me to have a glass of water or a snack or even to remember important appointments. Setting reminders helps you stick to the time that you've allocated to a specific task without running late for appointments or deadlines.

We all know how difficult it can be to stay focused on one task, especially when it's something that you have little to no interest in. Research suggests that spending time on the things that you don't particularly enjoy first will help you manage your time more efficiently.

If you start off with something that you enjoy, you might finish it quickly and then feel as though you're on top of your time until the task that you don't enjoy comes around. Since you've spent so much time on the things that you enjoy, you might feel demotivated and either procrastinate or drag the time out much longer than it needs to be.

If you start with something that you don't like, you'll be motivating yourself with a kind of "reward." Knowing that you'll get to what you like as soon as this specific task is wrapped up will certainly get you going, which brings us to our next topic.

Avoiding Procrastination

The first thing that you need to know is that procrastinating does NOT mean that you're lazy. People might procrastinate because they feel as if they're under a lot of pressure. This may seem to be counterproductive, and it is, but it's still one of the most common reasons for procrastination.

Chatty Cathy is a term that describes a woman with ADHD who is always telling her friends stories. She may even be a daydreamer, a clever, shy teenager with a cluttered locker.

However, what happens when she grows up? What if her ADHD isn't diagnosed till she's a woman? Is her situation unique compared to that of men with ADHD?

ADHD in women has gotten less attention. Although there seem to be some distinctions in ADHD symptoms between men and women.

According to Stephanie Sarkis, PhD, a psychotherapist in Boca Raton, Florida, adults with ADHD have the same issues as the general population. She believes that males with ADHD have a higher rate of automobile accidents, school suspensions, drug abuse, and aggressiveness and behavioral difficulties than females with ADHD. Regardless of ADHD, men are more predisposed to these types of diseases in general.

Women with ADHD are more prone to develop eating disorders, obesity, low self-esteem, depression, and anxiety. However, they do exist in the general population. These challenges typically show themselves in numerous facets of their lives. According to Anthony Rostain, MD, professor of psychiatry and pediatrics at the University of Pennsylvania School of Medicine, males with ADHD may have issues in the workplace, such as being unable to accomplish things or growing irritated with subordinates too easily.

Kathleen Nadeau, PhD, clinical psychologist and director of the Chesapeake ADHD Center of Maryland in Silver Spring, says her female ADHD patients, particularly parents, come to her in a "constant state of overwhelm."

"Society has certain expectations that we place on women, and ADHD frequently makes them more difficult to accomplish," argues Nadeau. She mentions traditional female social duties. "At residence, women are meant to be the organizer, planner, and lead parent. Women are expected to understand birthdays and anniversaries, as well as do laundry and make notes of upcoming activities. All of this is difficult for someone with ADHD."

Women's responsibilities, including things such as family and work, may make it increasingly challenging to disguise or control ADHD. Although there are some things women may do to manage challenges. Nadeau recommends that you educate your relatives and friends about ADHD so that they can be more encouraging and set realistic expectations for you. When feasible, women should simplify their lives.

Reduce stress and duties, and agree with relatives and partners about taking on the most challenging jobs.

Hiring a professional planner or training with a coach can also help you acquire good organizing habits and procedures. Sarkis recommends hiring an assistant for 6 to 8 hours a week to do light cleaning, go through paperwork, and help organize things.

"I've had people tell me that it'll be too expensive, and it could be, but many with ADHD can't afford assistance," Sarkis adds.

Women's ADHD, according to Rostain, is frequently overlooked until college, when they begin to display a lack of personality and ego. They are at risk of being misled by a sorority or the hard drug scene. Both struggle with organization, planning, knowledge retention, and paying attention.

Gender inequalities in ADHD symptoms, on the other hand, commonly occur. And the reason for this is most probably societal. By the time they reach maturity, the gap has narrowed to two to one. This is most probably since women are diagnosed later on in life than men.

Others might feel as if the upcoming task is not within their abilities. This mostly isn't the case at all. As you know, when it comes to women, this is a real concern. Some people simply say that they work better under more pressure, usually stated after they forget the intense stress and anxiety that comes with working too close to a deadline.

The first thing you can do to avoid this is to set deadlines for yourself. Or in other words, daily goals. Breaking up your work into smaller pieces might not only help time management but might also help you avoid procrastination. It's easy to become overwhelmed with a lot of work. Setting smaller goals for yourself will help you feel as if the load on your shoulders is lighter than you initially thought.

I find myself doing this all the time. When I work on a book, I feel overwhelmed because of all the work that still needs to be done. As soon as I start breaking the book into chapters and even sections within those chapters, I immediately feel relieved.

The next tip that I would like to share is to not try to do too many things at once. It's hard enough for us to concentrate and stay motivated with one project, never mind multiple. Multitasking might be something that gets associated with women all the time, but it's not something that a woman with ADHD should frequent.

You want to avoid failure, or the feeling of failure. In order to do that, you need to take things slowly and realize that it might take you longer than it would take others and that that's *okay*! It's also a good idea to avoid overstimulation and to eliminate as many distractions as you can.

Personally, I just can't concentrate on my work if there is a television on somewhere in the house. I need silence and peace. If you're the same, don't be afraid to switch that TV off or to tell your partner to turn down his own volume! Even if you work in an office environment, you can still politely ask your colleagues to be considerate. At the end of the day, your work is your income and it's important to give it your all.

It can be frustrating to have to work in situations that are less than desirable. Many other things can frustrate us just as much, if not more. The average human being experiences frustration frequently throughout the week. We get to experience it daily! That brings us to the next topic of discussion.

Problem-Solving Skills to Avoid Frustration

Frustration can stem from many different situations. They can be at work, at home, with friends or family, or anywhere in between! Realize that feeling frustrated is okay and normal. How you react to your frustration is where the difference comes in.

To avoid conflict and regret, it's always a good idea to think before you speak. Take a few minutes to feel and recognize your emotions. I always find that taking a few deep breaths really helps me to calm down and put things into perspective. You could also try anger management 101: count to 10. Don't be afraid to leave the room for a while if you need to.

After you've calmed down, your head should feel more clear, and it's at this stage when you can go ahead and express your feelings calmly and kindly. This advice helps in other situations of conflict as well. Taking these steps should ensure that you handle most difficult situations with dignity.

There are four steps that you can follow to resolve other more serious conflicts that can be related to problem-solving skills.

- Take the time to understand the problem and why it's considered a problem.

- Devise a sustainable plan that you and whoever may be involved can commit to.

- Carry out the plan that you've devised to the best of your abilities.

- Look back at the happenings that led to the problem in the first place and learn from past mistakes.

Impatience, frustration, and anger are common emotions for women with ADHD, even if they may not act on it as aggressively. For this reason, it would be a good idea to learn how to regulate your emotions as best you can.

Regulating Your Emotions

Remember when I said that we feel emotions more intensely? Well, that's not always a bad thing. Yes, we feel anger and frustration so deeply that it can sometimes drive us to the edge. But we also feel love and joy just as deeply. We feel our emotions and we should embrace them, embrace life. It's good to not repress our natural reactions, but we also need to understand that some of our reactions can negatively affect ourselves and other people. Therefore, while we embrace ourselves, we still need to ensure that the reactions we have towards more negative situations are appropriate yet still accurate representations of how we feel.

Regulating our emotions doesn't mean that we censor ourselves to the point where we're back to bottling up our feelings. It just means that we deal with the overwhelming and ever-flowing river inside us in a way that benefits us and the people around us.

Emotional regulation can be achieved by following these next five steps:

- **Choose situations that limit negative emotions.** You control your life and your exposures, and if you feel like you don't want to be in situations that are difficult for you to handle, then you don't want to be. Choosing what situations you want to be put in is not always easy, but, when possible, avoid situations that you know won't be good for your emotional state.

- **Control what you can in a situation.**

- **Pay attention to the parts of other situations that make you feel like it's still bearable.**

- **Reevaluate the negative situations that upset you.** Putting some thought into why it upsets you and what you can do to better, might help you in the long run.

Treatment Strategies for Co-Occurring ADHD and Substance Use Disorders

> *"Wherever the art of medicine is loved there is also a love of humanity."* - Hippocrates

The medications for treating ADHD have several benefits. They assist women with ADHD in doing better at college and work by lowering symptoms of hyperactivity, impulsivity, and inattention. They also enhance connections with family and friends.

Diagnosing ADHD in Women with SUD

ADHD remains a clinical diagnosis in children and adults; no neuropsychiatric or laboratory tests are clinically useful in detecting ADHD. Clinical diagnosis of ADHD in women remains difficult, especially in patients with co-occurring SUD due to a lack of consensus on diagnostic criteria, symptoms overlapping with other mental illnesses, and the necessity for a retrospective diagnosis of childhood ADHD. The ADHD criteria in the Diagnostic and Statistical Manual of Mental Disorders (DSM-IV-TR) were designed for diagnosing ADHD in children and are now used to diagnose ADHD in adults as well, but the validity of the criterion set is contested.

It is difficult to diagnose ADHD in people who are actively using drugs or who have recently begun sobriety. Substance misuse has a variety of acute and chronic consequences that resemble the symptoms of mental diseases such as ADHD. Stimulant use, for example, can cause changes in attentional ability and activity level both during intoxication and recovery, and chronic marijuana use can cause attention deficiencies. Furthermore, many individuals are unable to identify recent periods of abstinence from substance use, making it difficult to distinguish between basic and substance-induced symptoms.

Although some experts advocate examining individuals after a duration of lengthy abstinence, in many circumstances, this is not practicable. A comprehensive clinical history of symptoms during previous times of abstinence or before the commencement of drug use issues is often the best possible tool for determining whether inattention and hyperactive symptoms are caused by a primary condition or are caused by substances. Symptoms that appear during times of active substance use are hard to understand, since a diagnosis of ADHD is improper if they occur only in the setting of active substance use. Also, clinical identification of ADHD in adults remains difficult due to a lack of agreement on diagnostic criteria, notably the need that symptoms be evident before the age of seven.

Therefore, because self-reported historical diagnoses of childhood ADHD in women tend to overdiagnose ADHD, a cautious approach should be maintained. When working with women with SUDs, a rational solution could be to consider ADHD likely if symptoms can be recognized as having been consistent from early adolescence, but unusual if the symptoms arose concurrently or subsequently to the development of the SUD. External information from family members or an examination of objective data (for example, school performance statistics) can be quite helpful in evaluating whether symptoms existed from childhood.

While a diagnosis of ADHD is primarily clinical, some organized tools and discussions can help in the examination of an individual for ADHD. A thorough clinical battery, such as one used in research, would also include, in regards to a comprehensive psychiatric discussion, the Structured Clinical Interview for DSM-IV (SCID) and the Conners Adult ADHD Diagnostic Interview for DSM-IV (CAADID), which systematically assesses adult women for both childhood and adult symptoms. However, in many healthcare situations, completing a SCID and CAADID is not practical. Another more realistic strategy would be to conduct a semi-structured consultation guided by the DSM-IV TR criteria for ADHD (i.e., review symptoms in criteria set with the patient). The DSM-IV SNAP checklist and the ADHD Rating Scale-IV can also be used to test for ADHD symptoms. In any scenario, it is critical to collect data from additional informants (for example, a partner, parent, or close friend) to fully understand the type and intensity of the symptoms, as well as their influence on the patient's performance.

Psychosocial Therapies For ADHD and Co-Occurring SUD

While medicine is the foundation of ADHD treatment, a range of psychosocial interventions can be used in conjunction with medication to improve the long-term management of this chronic illness. Unfortunately, little controlled research on psychosocial interventions for adults with ADHD has been conducted. Data on pediatric therapies are unlikely to be immediately applicable since those interventions primarily focus on parent training and, in some situations, demonstrate the minor additional effect of psychosocial treatment on patients taking stimulant medication.

Cognitive Behavioral therapy (CBT) has been demonstrated to be beneficial in treating adult ADHD symptoms. CBT modifications like systematic skills training or cognitive rehabilitation have also been demonstrated to be helpful. However, there is proof that difficulties, such as those associated with ADHD, are associated with low treatment retention in patients receiving CBT for SUD, implying that maintaining patients with cognitive issues in CBT-based SUD treatment is hard and that personalized treatment strategies may be required.

Coaching and behavior modification are two other behavioral therapies for ADHD that are utilized therapeutically but have not been examined in controlled studies in adults. Tutoring is a collaborative partnership between a client and a professional to create solutions for dealing with issues including procrastination, time management, and organization. Behavior modification is a strategy used mostly with children in which desired actions are positively reinforced to boost their frequency.

ADHD Clinical Treatment for Co-Occurring With SUD

The treatment of individuals with co-occurring ADHD and SUD necessitates a thorough assessment of symptom load and impaired functioning. Since ADHD symptoms (e.g., impulsivity, poor planning) will interfere with SUD therapy, and drug use will limit the efficacy of ADHD treatment, treating both illnesses concurrently is likely to be the best strategy.

When administering psychostimulant medication for ADHD in patients with SUD, it is critical to pay close attention to the clinical context and therapeutic limits. It should be openly communicated with the patient that the use of stimulant medicine includes an inherent risk of abuse and misuse and that if proof of such development emerges, the validity of stimulant usage will be reassessed. The importance of adhering to the prescribed drug plan should not be underestimated, and medicine should not be used on an "as needed" basis. It should be made plain to the patient, and ideally, the family, that if it is discovered that prescription stimulant medicine is being misused, abused, or diverted, the physician is under no responsibility to continue therapy.

Fortunately, stimulant drugs may be rapidly withdrawn without serious consequences.

Psychostimulant usage in people with drug use disorders necessitates close supervision, including urine toxicological analysis. Recurrent or worsened drug usage may require re-evaluating the efficacy of the stimulant medication. All prescriptions must be meticulously documented to track the quantity and frequency of the substance being prescribed. Repeated demands to replace "missing," "lost," or "stolen" medicine, as well as comparable requests for dose increases that are not clinically substantiated, should be cause for worry. Postponed preparations are chosen because they lower the pace of change to drug blood levels, which is less encouraging, and they prevent non-oral usage. Client visits should be scheduled regularly.

Even with all mechanisms in place to minimize the risk of stimulant distraction, misuse, or abuse, it should also be anticipated that a minority of patients with ADHD who are also suffering from substance use disorders will engage in such nontherapeutic use, and that thorough clinical supervision will detect such nontherapeutic use slightly earlier and reduce its negative effects.

Rating instruments, such as the Conners Adults Attention-Deficit Rating Scale, might be useful for tracking symptom intensity over time and in response to withdrawal or ADHD medication. One key caution is that ADHD rating scales applied to individuals who have not completed a sustained period of abstinence will capture substance-induced symptoms of inattention and hyperactivity in addition to suspected ADHD symptoms. In such circumstances, using a sequential rating scale over time might assist in resolving the diagnosis; substance-induced symptoms would improve with withdrawal, whereas ADHD symptoms would be stable in the lack of therapy. Rating scales can offer standards against which the success of treatment can be assessed, especially when numerous pharmaceutical trials are necessary to produce a treatment diagnosis.

Given that stimulants, which are potentially addictive, are the basis of ADHD therapy, assessing for malingering is a crucial component of managing a patient with co-occurring ADHD and SUD. As lack of concentration symptoms dominate in women with ADHD and symptom evaluation is nearly entirely reliant on self-report, there is always the possibility of individuals with substance use disorders attempting to deceive physicians to receive stimulants. Efforts should be made to gather collateral data from relatives and other resources, including childhood school records.

Fidget Gadgets for Women With ADHD

Fidget gadgets, according to Dr. Pillar Trelles of the Icahn School of Medicine at Mount Sinai in New York City, "provide a less hazardous method to waste nervous energy." Fidget gadgets, such as stress balls and fidget spinners, reduce anxiety caused by ADHD by 18% and pain by 22%.

However, Dr. Trelles notes that the success of fidget toys is dependent on the sort of individual utilizing them. While anxiety, autism, ADHD, and other psychiatric illnesses exist on a continuum, so will the effectiveness of any fidget. Fidget toys, however, are a pleasant method to relax and keep calm and focused, regardless of your scenario.

Fidget toys are often intended to assist youngsters with anxiety and concentration issues. There is yet to be a definitive study on the influence of these toys, but early research indicates that they considerably improve children's attitudes, attentiveness, peer interactions, and writing ability.

There hasn't been much study done on the advantages of fidget toys for women. Nevertheless, many people who tried them indicate that they are effective in reaching a sense of calm. As a result, they help an individual's job productivity.

Are you ready to discover the greatest fidget toys for adult women? Let's get started!

- **Sculpture Building Blocks: Adult Stress Relief Toy**

This stress reliever toy serves two functions: stress alleviation during working hours and home furnishings. It comes with a 5 mm set of

1,000 construction magnets that will put your patience and ingenuity to the test. You have no restrictions on how you can create and decorate shapes and buildings.

This fidget toy is a wonderful device for both men and women that may improve your brain and inventiveness. If you are enamored of geometric patterns, it is most definitely the right toy for your concerns and anxiety. Due to the ease with which the little individual balls can be swallowed, keep it away from children and pets aged 13 and under.

- **Tangle Jr. Original Fidget Gadget**

The Tangle Jr. is available in three distinct hues, all of which are vivid and lively. You may combine them all to make your game more engaging and entertaining. It is advised for both adults and children, especially those who want to disconnect and get rid of technological devices.

Tangles are designed to keep your hands occupied while you are doing nothing. They are based on the principle of constant movement, which gives the mind and body a relaxing experience. You'll be able to create a variety of patterns once you start experimenting with them. As a result, your creativity and imagination will be boosted.

- **Toys Chuchik Fidget Cube**

Chuchik's wooden fidget gadget is ideal for individuals who wish to stay focused and far less distracted at work or college. It is generally marketed as a stress and anxiety reliever, but it also alleviates the symptoms of autism, ADD, ADHD, and OCD. You may play with it anyplace and at any time because it is compact and portable.

This toy may be used for a variety of purposes. You can roll, flip, spin, click, and glide. It relaxes tension and lessens irritability, in addition to relieving stress and boosting focus. If your mind becomes agitated, simply fidget with this fidget toy and you'll be able to find serenity in an instant.

- **Titanium Spinning Top by ForeverSpin**

Spinning tops are intended to improve your concentration and creativity. They keep your mental process and productivity going, especially if you're sitting at your desk. This ForeverSpin fidget spinning gadget is a sophisticated item that will complement your well-organized workspace.

You may push yourself to beat your spin times to make your game more enjoyable and engaging. You can also challenge your friends for whoever can spin the top the longest.

Spinning tops not only give relaxation and tranquility, but they also increase in-hand handling and hand-eye coordination.

- **Fidget Toy Infinity Cube**

This Small Fish offering is appropriate for both children and adults. It is an excellent method for releasing tension and relieving anxiety and stress. If you're looking for a toy to help you with your nail-biting, leg-shaking, as well as other fidgeting difficulties, this is the gadget for you.

In addition to its fidgeting advantages, this cube toy may increase the flexibility of your fingers. It can help you improve your fine motor abilities. It may be used anywhere, at any time, whether at work while thinking or at class while listening.

- **Flippy Chain Fidget Toy by Tom's Fidgets**

This chain fidget gadget is available in a variety of colors. It is constructed of stainless steel, which separates the rings and connects the chains without weakening or shattering. This product will help you quit smoking, manage anxiety and stress, and relieve tension at gatherings or events.

The Tom's Fidgets Flippy Chain is marketed as a "quiet yet gratifying" toy. The maker is proud of the product's unobtrusive quality. You may fidget and play as much as you like without garnering too much notice from others around you.

- **Crazy Aaron's Scarab Thinking Putty**

Crazy Aaron's product does not dry out easily because it is made of safe and non-toxic silicone. It comes in a variety of colors, shapes, and scents. It may be stretched, bounced, torn, or sculpted in any manner you wish.

While this medication is intended for younger adult women, it may also be used to ease tension in adult women. According to the company, it improves awareness, attention, and concentration. Its primary goal is to aid intelligence.

- **Fidget Cube Pilpoc theFube**

This fidget cube is composed of durable plastic and features squishy silicone rubber buttons. It is generally played with clicks, but if you are in a conference or a lecture, you could always turn off the sound. It's also highly portable, so you can carry it with you everywhere you go.

There are 12 sides of the product, each having a distinct fidget activity. Consider this Pilpoc item when you want to be relaxed and calm, or if you want to boost your attention and concentration.

- **Sensory Finger Rings That Are Spiky**

This is a unique fidget gadget that is a nice alternative to the standard ones. You move it back and forth between your fingers. The device is built entirely of high-quality stainless steel, making it suitable for both adults and suitably aged children.

These spiky finger rings are great for massaging as well as stress alleviation. Acupressure aids in the movement of good energy throughout the body. It also helps in the treatment of depression, discomfort, and sickness.

- **Fidget With Stretchy String**

These fidget strings are non-toxic and hypoallergenic. They do not include hazardous substances such as bisphenol A (BPA), phthalates, or latex. They are available in a variety of colors and can range from 10 inches to 8 feet.

You may bend, pull, spin, wrap, and squeeze these strings to satisfy your fidgeting needs. Then, enjoy seeing them revert to their normal shape. These fidget gadgets promote relaxation, decrease anxiety, and improve attention.

Chapter 4:

Dealing With Different Situations and Settings

Different settings may evoke different emotions and struggles that can make life more difficult than it needs to be. While it's important to be able to deal with the most common issues that we face every day, there are individual issues that relate to different environments such as your home life, work, social life, etc.

Dealing With Daily Struggles in Different Environments

Occupational Setting

Firstly, many of us might find it difficult to relate to the people we work with. This can lead to conflict and other problems; therefore, problem-solving skills are essential. There are multiple steps that can help you, but here are seven steps that you can focus on at first.

- Identify the conflict or problem: You need to fully grasp why there is conflict or why there is a problem, and exactly what those are.

- Understand the interests of every person involved.

- List the possible solutions to the problem as suggested by all involved parties.

- Evaluate the possible options.

- Choose an option or multiple options that everyone agrees on.

- Keep a document of the agreement.

- Agree on the future monitoring and the possible evaluation of progress.

These steps will help you deal with the more intense conflicts that may arise in your workplace. Let's talk about other kinds of conflicts that relate more to the internal aspects of yourself.

Communication can be difficult for people with ADHD. Some have suggested that we shouldn't really tell people that we have ADHD at work, as this can be seen as an excuse for why we can't perform as well as we should be able to for our positions. I believe that it's not a bad thing to let your superiors know that you have this condition, as long as you ensure that you do your absolute best to excel in your position. Ask for regular feedback in order to improve.

Organization is key for a clear mind. You've probably all seen the "memes" on social media. "ADHD means going insane amongst the disorganization but being too overwhelmed to organize." It's a feeling that most of us are aware of. You struggle to focus when things aren't organized or your workspace isn't tidy, yet you might lack the motivation to do something about it and when you eventually do, it doesn't take long for disorganization to set in again.

So, it kind of feels like unavoidable turmoil, but it doesn't have to be. We've already established that your concentration will be much more effective if your space is tidy and your things are organized. The good news is that this might be your wake-up call that will spark the motivation to do something about it. The bad news is that the motivation might not last very long.

How can you ensure that you stay motivated enough to see this plan through and keep it that way? Well, it's not as difficult as it may sound. Every person is different, and therefore, not every piece of advice will work for everyone, but it could be as simple as setting smaller goals for yourself. I've mentioned this before, and I'd like to mention it again because it truly does help in so many different situations.

In this situation, you might feel overwhelmed by all the organizing that lies ahead of you. To combat this feeling, you can break the space up into sections. Let's say you have a whole office to work on. Start with your desk. You can work on one of your bookshelves the next day, maybe one drawer at a time for the next day. Whatever works for you.

Leaving positive notes for yourself around your office or even your house might help you stay motivated as well. "Be wise, organize!" is probably the phrase I write on every note that I leave for myself around my space. It really helps!

How do you keep the newly organized sections from falling into chaos again? Well, you can add stickers to every drawer or shelf with the names of what you want to store there written on them. This will remind you where everything is supposed to go. Reminding yourself to put it back there doesn't have to be difficult, either. It might sound silly, but I have found that labeling most of my things with "put me back" stickers have really helped! My husband even started writing the phrase on the milk because I always leave it out.

Another part of dealing with work settings is to be mindful of your time management. Since you have some helpful tips on how to manage your time now, you should be able to implement these tips in your workplace as well. Time management should help relieve some of the stress and anxiety that goes with a busy schedule.

Another helpful tip for both time management and work-related issues would be to prioritize your tasks and appointments. For example, a task that has a deadline coming up in a week might need to be prioritized over a task that you still have a whole month to prepare for.

This doesn't only relate to specific tasks and appointments; you can also prioritize your entire day and all the little things that go with it. You might need to head to the nail salon soon, but you might also need time to rest and reflect. While both of these would be considered self-care, having an hour or two to rest might be in your best interest. It all depends on your personal schedule and the things that are more important to you and your well-being.

Mind Your Mouth

I don't know about you, ladies, but my personality can be a bit on the rebellious side. In my research, I have found that a lot of women with ADHD have the same issue. It's not always an issue, and having a strong personality can be a good thing if it means that you don't let people walk all over you yet still remain calm and professional. The way I see it, women with ADHD tend to be either completely submissive and reserved or completely aggressive and rebellious. I'm sure there are women who fall somewhere in the middle, but I have yet to meet them.

We need to strive to be in the middle. Standing firm in our moral values and ambitions, yet giving way for constructive criticism and following orders when necessary. Unless you're lucky enough to play the "boss" role, you probably need to take orders from someone daily. This is something that I struggle with all the time, the little rebel in me fights back viciously when I am *told* to do something and not politely asked.

In all honesty, not every person in a position of authority will have the people skills that they actually need. They won't all be kind and thoughtful, and they won't all be polite enough to ask certain things of us instead of demanding them. In all my years, I have learned that this isn't something we can change. Instead, for your own benefit, you should try to let it slide past you as much as you can while still letting your feelings be known in a professional way.

We work to put food on the table and to be able to buy that pretty dress or pair of jeans that we've been eyeing, not to make friends or to get into arguments with authority. Everything that you do at work is for your own benefit. You'd much rather be known as a team player than as someone who can't be relied on. This isn't about what people think of you, but rather about the benefits or opportunities that may come from doing your part and more.

My point? Don't let people walk over you or take advantage of you, but learn when to simply let things slide for the greater good and when to follow directions.

Distractions

As you now know, distractions need to be eliminated. When you're at work, it would be a good idea to switch your phone off unless you need it for set reminders or for work. You can switch the volume off and set a timer to check it once an hour if you think that it may help.

If you're worried about emergencies, you can politely ask your friends and family to not contact you during work hours unless it's an emergency. It might also be helpful to wear some soundproof ear gear, depending on how serious your need for silence is.

Tips for a Short Memory Span

The best advice that I can give here is to always take notes and to record important meetings if your company doesn't have any kind of policy against that sort of thing. You can also follow up conversations with an email (Hurley, 2016). This will help to clarify any kind of misunderstandings that might have occurred.

Hyperactivity

Some of us find it more difficult to be confined to a desk for long periods; therefore, short body breaks are the best thing that you can do to combat hyperactivity. Stand up regularly and stretch your legs, wiggle your hips, maybe even twist your fingers around.

You can also keep a stress ball close by. These don't only help with stress, they're also rather fun to mess around with when you feel fidgety. I found that keeping a bit of clay in my hand while working was a great way to help me concentrate and to keep me from shaking my desk around with my legs.

Homelife

Many of the tips I have given so far should help you at home as well, but there are a few things that relate more to your home than they would to anything else. Let's talk about organizing and decluttering your house.

- **Decluttering Your House**

You might be wondering what I mean by clutter. Clutter refers to anything that you choose to keep that you don't use anymore or that you haven't used in a long time. Basically, anything that does not add more value or worth to your life.

When it comes to women who have ADHD, extra clutter is a sure way to add extra stress. We tend to want to hold on to things that offer no value and the results are hours of looking for things that we need daily. All the clutter could make organizing and staying on top of your schedule seem more difficult than it should be.

If you want to feel more in control and relaxed, we need to get rid of all the clutter!

Here are some examples of what clutter could be:

- Clothes that don't fit

- Old toys that haven't been played with in years

- Excess tupperware

- Excess cutlery and other kitchen items

- Old empty perfume bottles that were gifts

- Empty gift bags

- Old makeup products

- Empty wrappers and plastic bags

- Old baby things

- Tools that aren't being used

- Old hair accessories

It's easy to start hoarding clothes. As we get older, our bodies change all the time. You might be keeping clothes that are too small for you, hoping that you'll fit into them again. You might be afraid to gain an excessive amount of weight and keep clothes that are too big for you. You might even be keeping clothes that you simply don't wear anymore because you never thought to get rid of them.

Keeping clothes that don't fit you can be incredibly demotivating and bad for your self-esteem. There are multiple organizations that would be happy to receive donated clothes for the less fortunate. Understandably, some people don't like donating to organizations. If this is the case for you, you can give the clothes to individual people that you know need them.

Similarly, old toys and baby things can be donated to organizations or individual people who might have more use for them than you. Most old makeup products should probably be discarded, but I have fond memories of my mother passing on her old eyeshadow palettes to me for dress-up play when I was a girl. It depends on your own opinions. Either way, they need to go.

Some people keep drawers full of plastic bags and wrappers. These clutter your things and they're bad for your environment. They should be discarded in a safe and suitable way.

Most of the items on the list are things that can easily be passed on or thrown away. Don't let sentimental value turn into hoarding. The relief and sense of accomplishment that goes with decluttering is worth every sad goodbye to every old throw pillow or china doll!

Here are some general tips on how you can declutter your home:

- Plan your steps and where you want to discard the items or who you want to donate them to.

- Don't try to declutter the whole house in one day. Take your time and do it step by step.

- When sorting, you can still keep a few sentimental things. For example, your late mother's broaches or other similar things. But pack them away neatly and store them where they won't get in the way of your daily items.

- Label different boxes with things in them to prevent any misunderstandings. You wouldn't want to accidentally donate your most frequently used items.

- Consider a garage sale if some of your items can't be donated or if you're a little short on cash.

Decluttering is a personal experience and there is no right or wrong way to do it, as long as the results are the same.

- **Organizing Your Home**

After you've gotten rid of all the unnecessary items, you will already feel a giant load lifted from your shoulders. As soon as the last box leaves the front door, it's time to… take a well-deserved break and have a glass of wine (or juice). You'll deserve some rest after this ordeal! Decluttering is said to be both physically and mentally exhausting, but at least you'll burn a few extra calories.

The next step is to organize your house and the items that you've decided to keep. It's also important to plan ahead for a way to not fall into disorganization again. Tips previously mentioned will aid you in this quest.

I've gone and researched this topic extensively, and there is one article that I came across that offered amazing tips that I'll be sharing here today. The article is by Amanda Garrity, and it was published in June of 2021 on the *Good Housekeeping Home* website.

The first organizing tip relates more to your kitchen. Garrity suggests vertical shelves for cutting boards and other items. Not everyone will have the opportunity to change their shelving, but for those of you who do, I have to admit that it makes it much easier to get to things without having to cause a mess. I often used to have to pack everything out of the pots and pans cupboard in order to find a specific pan until I gave vertical shelves a shot!

Compartmentalizing your drawers will also prevent disorganization to set in once you've finished organizing. Keep similar things together and be sure to label them to remind you to put everything back where it belongs.

Your kitchen can be organized in whatever way suits you. If you have a pantry, you can organize it starting from fruits and vegetables, all the way to spices and pasta. Arrange it to make the things that you eat most frequently more easily accessible. It might also be a good idea to keep breakfast goods together while keeping ingredients for lunch and dinner in separate areas.

Depending on what your line of work is, Garrity suggests having a specific closet that's dedicated to your work things. You can organize the cupboard alphabetically and keep all your books and files in a tidy little workspace. She also suggests installing a space-saving desk. These are mounted to the wall and can be set up when you need it and put away when you're done.

Your linen closet can sometimes be an endless pit of rags, so be sure to donate the things that you really don't use often. You can start by folding the face cloths and face towels in one area and packing the closet from left to right. Garrity suggests adding towel railings to the linen closet door. This is a pretty creative idea that might make access to towels easier and it'll also save some space!

When it comes to most of your hair care products or any other smaller items around the house, you'll spare yourself a lot of hassle by simply adding plastic bins to the walls or cabinet doors in order to store these items.

I think this next tip is great. Garrity suggests hooking two hangers together by using a can tab. This way, you can save closet space and hang more clothes! I couldn't believe that I never thought about it and now, all my hangers are double!

If you have an old wardrobe in the garage, you can consider painting the old drawers and slipping them under your bed. This way, you'll have more storage space (neatly organized) without using more space in the bedroom(s).

Another interesting suggestion was to hang your jewelry on a pegboard (Garrity, 2021). You can organize them from favorite to least favorite. With easy access and an easy enough way to put them back after using them, there's no way that your jewelry will fall into disorganization again.

If you have a partner with a messy space full of tools, you'll want to get them in on the action, too! Keeping your house organized means that you'll need to get everyone in the game as well. All your hard work won't mean a thing if it only lasts a few days.

For children, you can try using a reward system; for some partners, this method may be effective, too (wink wink). Leaving sticky notes as reminders around the house might help in this situation as well. The most important thing you can do is to speak to your family and let them know how important it is for you and your mental health.

Here's an extra tip: If you're anything like me, then chances are, you frequently misplace your things. Keeping the house organized should help with that. If you can remind yourself to put things back where they go, they're less likely to go missing. Unless, of course, you have little gremlins running around with your stuff all day (Ah, motherhood).

Creating a Cleaning Schedule With a Checklist

You've made it this far! Gone is the clutter and disorganization! Now, it's time to create a cleaning schedule to help you keep it this way! For me, it's better to know that I have a schedule and a checklist to stick to, as this ensures that I don't miss anything and that I stay motivated!

The lists I have that work for me are as follows:

- Daily
- Weekly
- Monthly

Okay, before you skip this section because it sounds like too much work, let me tell you that it's easier than it looks. You might feel a little intimidated by taking on these responsibilities and staying on top of this kind of organizing. That's perfectly normal, and I want you to stop doubting yourself because you can do this.

I am plagued by intimidating tasks all the time; we all are. But if you close your eyes and push through, you might be surprised by what you can accomplish!

I am going to give you some examples of checklists that you can customize for your own home and situation.

Daily Checklist

	Dishes/ bathrooms cleaned	Sweep	Wipe counters	Dust	Pick up toys
Morning	x	x	x	x	x
Afternoon	N/A	N/A	N/A	N/A	N/A
Evening	x	x	x	x	x
	Mom/Dad	Peter	Jackson	Maddie	Lilly

This sample list shows you how simple it can be to keep your home neat and tidy during the day. Each family member is given one or two tasks (depending on how many people there are in the family). When you break it up like this, it doesn't seem so intimidating anymore.

Don't be afraid to let older kids help out with dishes, too. My daughter was six years old when I first started letting her help out with them. At first, you can stick around to help the older child and teach them which things to wash first. As they learn, you can start leaving them to it while you take care of different chores.

You should try to avoid letting your kids feel overwhelmed with chores, as they can feel just as we do when it comes to this kind of work. You don't want them cleaning all day, every day. That's why a good rule to follow is twice a day, depending on your personal needs, and it might only be necessary for certain chores once a day.

A house with many children and a lot of people will need the dishes done more than once a day, and toys will need to be picked up more than once as well. So you can really go and assess the needs of your home and create your list according to that.

You could also add taking care of pets to the list if you have them. It's good for children to learn to take responsibility for their pets. They can feed them and give them clean water as an extra chore.

Weekly Checklist

Saturdays (Any day you prefer)	Wash bed linen and other laundry/ cut the grass/clean the grill	Mop the floors/make sure Mom has all the lunch boxes/vacuum cleaning	Sweep the porch/water the plants	Clean the windows/wash inside of the kitchen cabinets	Dust the bookshelf/wash inside of the fridge	Arrange the toys neatly/ensure that school uniforms are ready
	x	x	x	x	x	x
	x	x	x	x	x	x
	x	x	N/A	N/A	N/A	N/A
Mom/Dad	Jackson	Peter	Maddie	Lilly	All kids	

In this sample, the family spring cleans the house once a week. Sometimes you may want to go away for the weekend or the kids might visit a friend, and in this case, they can do their weekly chores on a different day (as long as it gets done at some point). When the whole family is away or if the weekly chores don't get done for some other reason, it can always be skipped until the next week. It's not the end of the world, but daily chores will ensure the relative tidiness of the home.

Having a checklist and schedule doesn't mean that you can't have a life and that it's life or death if something gets skipped. It's just a general guideline for families who have trouble with keeping up. If you're lucky enough to have some paid help around the house, then you can still give your kids simple chores to help out with to teach them to take responsibility for themselves and their messes.

In this case, kids can still pick up toys and look after their pets. You can have a mini checklist for their rooms that can help them remember what to do, like making the bed and putting their clean laundry away.

Monthly Checklist

Curtains washed/garage cleaned	Walls washed	All pets bathed	Neatly arranged closets	Neatly arranged closets
x	x	x	x	x
Mom/Dad	Peter	Jackson	Maddie	Lilly

Monthly chores are the kinds of chores that you don't worry about too often but that still need to be done in order to ensure proper hygiene. Again, every household is different, and your lists may look very different from these sample lists. It may seem like a lot of work, but with everyone pitching in, you'll see just how quickly it can go!

This is a simple and efficient suggestion to get your whole family involved in the upkeep of your home. This helps women with ADHD in the sense that they don't feel that the whole house balances on their shoulders, because it shouldn't. This is the 21st century, and women don't take care of their homes alone anymore.

Whenever you feel overwhelmed, don't forget to take a breather on your own for a minute. It's not selfish to want five minutes to collect yourself. In fact, I encourage it.

Parenthood

So many people don't realize how much it really takes from us, from any woman. Having a job, a family, and a home to care for is no easy task. Especially not when you have ADHD. Intense emotions, lack of concentration, and memory loss can make dealing with daily life feel more overwhelming than it needs to be.

The fact is, you don't have to be perfect all the time; nobody is. You don't have to beat yourself up for what you consider to be mistakes, and you don't have to compare yourself to anyone else. There will always be some perfect mom with a perfect family on social media. In reality, she probably has just as many bad days as you do.

- **Explaining your condition to family members** might help solve a lot of conflicts. Your loved ones won't understand your symptoms unless you explain it to them. You can then work together on how to solve possible problems.

Awareness is key in this situation; the last thing we need is for people who don't understand what we have to face daily criticizing us on our parenting or even our homes. Sometimes it might feel as if your partner and children demand more from you than you can give. While your partner might understand, children likely won't. To them, you are Mom. Caregiver, doctor, psychologist, chef, and friend.

- **Taking enough time for yourself will be very necessary.** Even when your workday ends, the work at home never seems to. So, go ahead and get a babysitter now and again! Even if it's just the kids visiting Grandma for an evening while you take a hot bath.

- **You can also wake up a little earlier** than your family in the mornings. I have been doing this for years, and my most precious time is my alone time before the chaos erupts. This time allows you the chance to get your thoughts together and to review your schedule. It also gives you that extra breather that every mother needs.

It doesn't have to be a whole hour or more before the kids wake up; 15 minutes to half an hour should do the trick. There was a time when I would set my alarm for a whole two hours earlier in order to do my makeup and get myself as ready as possible. It felt great to be able to take my time, but it also cut my sleep cycle much shorter. For this reason, I decided to make it 30 minutes. No more, no less.

- **Be sure to do as much as you can to avoid chaos in the mornings.** We all know the feeling; the day has barely started and everyone is already shouting. You can do this by making sure that you set clothes out and pack lunch boxes the evening before.

- **Letting your children help out around the house** can be a fun way of lessening the burden on your shoulders. This works better for older children. Some moms might feel like it would create more chaos or that they would feel annoyed at half-done chores. Others feel like it helps relieve stress and creates opportunities for bonding. Whatever you decide is perfectly fine. Give it a try before dismissing the idea, though.

- This tip is a rule that should help most mothers, whether ADHD is present or not. **You should try being as consistent with rules and routines** as much as you possibly can. This will help your children follow their routines more easily, which should make your life easier. When you feel overwhelmed with emotions and frustration, it can be tempting to let something "slide." Here's the thing, though; the more you let things "slide," the more difficult it becomes to enforce those rules or any rules at a later time.

- While we don't want to let too many things "slide," we also need to **be mindful of the things that may not be worth the fight.** A good example of this might be a child who seems to be a picky eater. Some moms would disagree with me, but I feel like we shouldn't force children to eat something that they truly dislike. As adults, we have our likes and dislikes, too. That doesn't mean that we'll be filling them full of candy instead of food.

In fact, if you're a mom with ADHD, then there is a chance that your children, or at least one of them, might have it, too. For this reason, it might be better to steer clear of sugary candies and chocolates for the first few years. When I was a child, a doctor recommended to my mother that I have very small amounts of sugar at a time to prevent the worsening of hyperactivity and other symptoms.

As a mother, I have to agree. I've seen it in my own kids. We want to lessen our struggles and prevent conflict, and having kids jumping from the walls for hours is definitely not a way to do that.

- Along with explaining to your partner all about your condition, it would be helpful if **they could be more involved with the kids as well**. Your partner is called your partner for a reason, and this means that they need to be ready to take over when you feel as if your frustration or anger can't be contained for much longer.

Mothers With ADHD Raising a Child With ADHD

Parenting a child with ADHD is not for the faint-hearted, and it becomes much more difficult when you, too, struggle to remain on track every day. Nonetheless, given the exceptionally high heritability rates for this perplexing condition, millions of moms with ADHD today confront this issue. According to research, ADHD is more heritable than most other mental illnesses, just slightly less so than height, resulting in a variety of colorful familial relationships.

According to Andrea Chronis-Tuscano, Ph.D., an associate professor of psychology at the University of Maryland, the burden of parenting a kid with ADHD is challenging for parents who have the same problem. Chronis-research Tuscano concentrates on this double combo— women with ADHD raising children with ADHD—making her completely aware of how blatantly inaccurate she was. "We've seen that parents with increased ADHD symptoms struggle to be positive and keep their emotions in check, while also being inconsistent in terms of discipline: they frequently say one thing and then do another. Distracted mothers also have difficulty closely watching their children, which may be dangerous considering how accident-prone children with ADHD are."

In several instances, ADHD-diagnosed parents and children might be a perfect mismatch. Parenting necessitates the use of the brain's executive functions, which include exercising excellent judgment, planning ahead of time, being patient, and remaining calm. When women who are battling with these issues have children who are also struggling, you're likely to have more project delays, general mistakes, emotional outbursts, and, just as frequently, profoundly humorous moments.

According to Chronis-Tuscano, she has had women come into her study for interviews, check their watches, and race off to pick up children who were waiting for them someplace else.

Liz Fuller, a housewife from Chandler, Arizona, understands what it's like. Fuller has two boys, one of which has ADHD as well as increased autism. Fuller has never been diagnosed with ADHD, but she believes she would have been if she had the opportunity to see a doctor.

She claims that now and again, she is the sole Mom attempting to bring her child to school on a day when school is not even in session. "Oops, if it wasn't written down, it mustn't be true," she quips. She often forgets from time to time that she had already sent her child to a disciplinary time-out and, even more frequently, forgets why he is being placed there.

Fuller, who used to work in a commercial human resource department, has discovered that full-time parenting is significantly more difficult than college or the working world. In contrast to these other hobbies, motherhood, she observes, provides "no formula or structure," resulting in circumstances in which "you are gazing at a million diversions and tasks to do, and none of this can be tucked in a manila folder for later."

As Fuller attempted to keep a reward chart for her seven-year-old to urge him to switch off his video game at night when his time was up, she was frequently too preoccupied with putting her other two children to bed to notice the "teachable moments" when he cooperated. At times, she acknowledges that she completely forgot she was maintaining the charts.

While some situations might be amusing, the repercussions of a double diagnosis are not so. Researchers discover a greater likelihood of divorce and drug misuse issues among parents of children with ADHD, whereas mothers of children with ADHD report greater levels of melancholy and a sense of social exclusion than mothers parenting children without the disorder.

Melanie Salman, a part-time event organizer in the San Francisco Bay Area and a mother of two, is still upset over what transpired at her New Year's Eve event. Her pals had decided to build a small image of a political person they all despised and burn it at midnight. Right as they were about to burn it, her nine-year-old son, who has ADHD, came to Salman and said, "Hey, Mom, if I was going to build a doll to burn, it would be you!"

"I couldn't help but think about how, despite working with a psychologist, pediatrician, occupational therapist, and cognitive-behavioral psychologist, as well as a learning resources team, his school teachers, and music teachers, while also smoothing over his attitude with friends and exercising him like a puppy to calm him down," Salman wrote me in an email.

The image of her seven-year-old daughter wailing after she could not even find her mother at midnight, she adds, made it far worse. "I held her, apologized, and sobbed because I realized I had been so concentrated on the negative that I had forgotten to enjoy the positive and joy in my life."

This leads us to the good side of the double knot. After going through it for over seven years, she is certain that the more self-awareness you bring towards this turmoil and difficult scenarios, the more it may wind up being a spiritual adventure. You can thank your child someday if you can survive it.

In a study published in *Development and Psychopathology*, Lamprini Psychogiou, Ph.D., a lecturer and researcher at the University of Exeter in the United Kingdom, gives a positive picture of the prospective results of a shared diagnosis. Psychogiou discovered in a study of over 300 mothers that, while ADHD symptoms in children were associated with more negative feelings exhibited by their mothers, women who matched their children's symptoms were far more loving and sympathetic.

Liz Fuller is one example of this mindset. Her favorite ADHD parenting tale takes place before her child got diagnosed with ADHD. She was distraught because he was the only toddler in his music class who just couldn't sit still in the ring. Later that same day, Fuller took a shower—so preoccupied, as always, that she shampooed her hair twice. She had forgotten whether she had shaved her legs. She screamed in rage as she just remembered the other moms' looks as she chased him all around the room and murmured warnings in his ear.

However, Fuller recalls her turbulent upbringing, noting how frequently she was suspended in junior high for disruptive conduct, such as conversing with other students and being unable to remain quiet. "I had this good understanding of my son for the first time," she recalls. "He couldn't say much, but he was telling me a lot with his actions. He didn't want (or need) to sing in a circle. He wasn't attempting to offend or irritate me. He was uninterested! I, for one, was bored. Who likes sitting in a ring and listening to other children sing songs whenever there is work to be done? And who wants to have a child sit in a ring?"

Fuller dropped out of the music class in favor of keeping frequent play dates with her child in the park, where "we strolled freely and explored the wonderful outdoors, where we are both happiest, anyhow."

A mother with ADHD parenting a child with ADHD is a superhero. Even with all the ups and downs, there will always be a silver lining.

Relationships

Relationships can be incredibly difficult when you have ADHD. You might constantly feel as if you're being criticized, nagged, or micromanaged (Smith, 2019). If your ADHD has been diagnosed and you're being treated, the problems will likely be less severe, although not non-existent.

To those of you reading this book because of a loved one who has ADHD and not yourself, I understand that you might often feel lonely or ignored (Smith, 2019). There is an explanation for this, as women who struggle with ADHD can sometimes struggle with communication, which further puts pressure on a relationship.

- As a young woman, my previous partner felt underappreciated and ignored when I "zoned out" during conversations or if I forgot little things that he might have previously mentioned. The more I tried explaining that I couldn't help it, the more he got frustrated and upset.

- That's an example of what you *don't* want in your relationship. There has to be mutual respect and a hell of a lot of patience in order for this kind of relationship to work. Regardless of how long you've been together, you need to consider putting yourself in your partner's shoes (Smith, 2019).

- Talk about your feelings and frustrations while remaining calm. The best advice that I can give is to really try to listen and understand how your partner is feeling. You might have a whole bunch of emotions running through your head, and your partner likely does, too. Even if the emotions that they're experiencing might be different.

- The more you know about ADHD, the less difficult it will be to realize its impact on the relationship and resolve the problems (Smith, 2019). Ask your partner to not take symptoms personally, remind them that your brain works differently than theirs does (Smith, 2019).

- Women who have ADHD often feel ashamed in their relationships, just as much as they do throughout daily life. Your relationship is supposed to be a safe space where feelings such as shame have no place. For your relationship to be fruitful and positively influenced, you need to let go of that shame and guilt. Negative feelings like these can cause resentment and anger in relationships, whether they're romantic or not.

- Make time for each other. With all the stress of home life and/or kids, among other things, it can be difficult to focus on the love and affection that's necessary for a bond to survive between two people. Focus on what brought you together in the first place. Date nights once every two or three weeks would be a great way to start.

It might help to find a little humor in different situations (Smith, 2019). It might not be funny at the time, but the sight of you looking for your cellphone while it's in your hand is funny. Don't be upset if a giggle escapes your partner. Use those silly moments to break the ice!

When it comes to family and platonic relationships, the struggles can be similar. The people who don't have the condition might feel as if the friendship or relationship is more one-sided. They might also feel many of the same emotions that a romantic partner would feel, such as being ignored or offended.

The fortunate aspect is that family members have spent a lot more time with you than most friends or romantic partners might have. That means that they probably understand a lot more about your symptoms and behavior. This doesn't refer to all the extended family, but your parents or siblings who grew up with you likely understand you more than you know.

Okay, it might feel a little offensive to have your friends, close family members, and partner chat about you, but it shouldn't be. It could be very helpful for them and you. Your partner and your close friends could receive helpful advice on how to deal with certain symptoms from your closest family members. It's all about being a team.

Social Skills and Social Anxiety

Unfortunately, there hasn't been much research on this topic, either. I did find an article that I felt was as helpful as it could be, under the circumstances. The article was posted in a magazine called *CHADD*. You can find the articles online as well. The site contains numerous helpful articles to help improve the lives of people with ADHD.

The article that I'll be sharing with you was titled "Relationships and Social Skills." According to the article, 50-60% of children with ADHD have trouble with social relationships. This can last into adulthood for reasons that I'm sure you must be well aware of by now.

Among the various tips and facts stated in the relationship, there are a few that stood out to me. They suggest paying close attention to conversations that might be of importance for your social life. When you have ADHD, it's easy to have momentary lapses of attention which could result in you missing crucial information. For example, if a friend asks you to meet them at the restaurant at 7 p.m., but you miss the "7 p.m." part, this could lead to frustration and misunderstandings.

It would be best to ensure that you confirm all times and places more than once to avoid conflict. When it comes to friendships, you'll need to show your loved ones that you care by also paying attention to details about themselves that they may share. To help you remember these, you could write them down in your journal as soon as you get a chance.

I once met a friend who wrote down my favorite colors, songs, food, everything. When I found his journal, I felt very appreciated and thankful. Since then, I have been making a point of doing the same. I write down what I might forget. Not only for reference later, but the act of writing it down makes it even easier to remember.

The article also suggests that you pay attention to the people around you for clues as to how you could possibly behave and how they're feeling. Body language is a huge indication of their true feelings. By watching facial expressions, hand gestures, and more, you can pinpoint how to react around the person or how to take the conversation further.

Impulsivity can have a very negative effect on your social life. Other people may not understand the behavior and attribute it to carelessness. It would be wise to explain to your friends, once again, that your symptoms are not always controllable and that it doesn't mean that you don't care. Tips previously mentioned about taking a moment to think before you act or speak will help in these situations as well.

When it comes to your social life, it's good to be yourself and to be honest and true, but some people might just not understand the true you. We also want to avoid unnecessarily offending people or hurting their feelings. None of us intend to do so, but impulsive behavior might still result in such. For this reason, we censor ourselves a little and truly reflect on the situations.

Whatever your situation is, there is always room for kindness. As the old saying goes, "If you can't say something nice, don't say anything at all."

Chapter 5:

Improving Your Focus

We've covered many tips on how to improve concentration and focus so far, but there are some tips that I felt needed more attention. As an adult woman with ADHD, your focus and concentration are of utmost importance for basically every daily task. Without the proper focus, your life could erupt into chaos.

This could follow from simple misunderstandings, such as a time or location, or big misunderstandings that could relate to your work or safety. Luckily, there are some fun ways in which you can improve your focus and concentration such as brain train games and more!

Games That Improve Your Focus

- **Sudoku**

This game first appeared in Japan in the late 1980s. It's a relatively popular game that people of all ages seem to enjoy. The game requires concentration and critical thinking (Raypole, 2019). The game is said to improve both concentration and memory. Working with numbers might not be for everyone, but you won't know unless you try!

- **Crossword Puzzles**

There are millions of fun crossword puzzles out there, and they are said to improve memory and concentration, although many experts believe this to be a myth. Either way, they still improve your vocabulary and intellect. I believe that they might still improve concentration because it takes concentration and critical thinking to find the proper words. Since it's educational and fun, give it a try anyway!

- **Chess**

This game goes without saying, but I'll say it anyway. There are so many benefits to a game of chess that it sticks out as one of the top games for brain training. Not only does it improve your focus, but it also improves problem-solving skills and more! There are even rumors that it might promote creativity by activating the right side of the brain.

Chess is also a great way to bond with friends and family, so you can train your brain while having family time! It's a win-win situation.

- Jigsaw Puzzles

Studies show that the physical act of putting puzzles together improves short-term memory, concentration, and problem-solving skills (DeBakey, 2020). Puzzles are also another great way to help relieve stress and anxiety and they also make for great bonding time with your loved ones! You can puzzle by yourself too if that works better for you.

The Importance of Sleep

It's no secret that getting enough sleep is crucial for your health, regardless of what conditions you may have. Whether it's your physical or mental health that you're looking to improve, sleep will be your friend. Adults need at least seven hours of uninterrupted sleep. For mothers, that's not always possible. This is why it's important to get as much sleep as you can, when you can.

Sleep deprivation can lead to worsening symptoms such as lack of concentration or focus. It may also affect your moods and emotions. For this reason, you need to work on your sleep schedule by setting a bedtime for yourself. It has also been suggested that you steer clear of phones and laptops for at least an hour before bedtime. These things might stimulate your brain, and we don't want that. We want the brain to ease down and rest.

If you find yourself struggling to sleep, there are a number of things you can try to improve this:

- Don't eat close to bedtime.

- Have a cup of tea about two hours before bedtime.

- Try white noise.

- Don't leave a television or radio on during the evening.

- Try stretching before bed.

- Don't have water too close to bedtime to eliminate bathroom trips throughout the night.

ADHD can impact your sleep negatively. People who have ADHD can often suffer from insomnia, and children who suffer from ADHD often also have trouble with nightmares. For others, ADHD might cause excessive sleeping, which also relates to underlying depression. ADHD can also lead to a racing mind! It's not just our bodies that can suffer from hyperactivity, our minds can, too, so follow some of the above tips to get your brain to "chill out" enough for you to fall asleep!

It's always best to consult with your healthcare practitioner about sleeplessness that you can't relieve with simple remedies. ADHD can also lead to trouble falling asleep, and some people describe the feeling as having an "overactive brain that just won't switch off." Depending on the severity of your situation, your doctor might prescribe medications to help you sleep.

The Benefits of Exercise

Every healthcare professional will tell you about how important and beneficial exercise is for any person. For various reasons, exercise has been recommended for people with ADHD for years. There are multiple benefits that relate to your physical and mental health. Exercise has also long been known to improve focus and concentration.

Let's look at some of the physical benefits first.

Benefits for Physical and Mental Health

Physical Health

Your heart health should be on the top of your priority list regardless of your age. Many younger people don't realize the damage that they cause during these years but feel the negative effects later in life.

Here are some benefits for your heart:

- Exercise improves your cholesterol.

- Could lower high blood pressure.

- It has also been suggested that it reduces the risk of heart disease and heart attacks.

- Might also reduce the risks of a stroke.

Regular exercise is also said to reduce the risk of certain cancers such as colon, stomach, uterine, breast, and kidney cancers (Daniels, 2021). Along with these obvious benefits, your fitness levels are also improved, which will lead to a better quality of life.

Regular exercise also helps you sleep better, which obviously benefits every aspect of your physical and mental health. It has been recommended that an adult should work out at least four times a week for at least 40-45 minutes. This amount of exercise should quickly show some results. Weight loss is another benefit that exercise may have, just be sure to remember that exercise alone will likely not help you to lose more than a few pounds. Healthy eating habits also need to be considered.

There has also been speculation about whether regular exercise can help you with clear skin. Some experts believe this to be so (Semeco, 2017). Another interesting benefit that I have proven to myself over and over again is that exercise aids digestion and might even be a good way of treating constipation. Feeling bloated? Hop on that treadmill!

Regular exercise will also improve bone health and muscle mass. As you get older, your muscles and bones are often the first parts of your body to feel your age. If you incorporate a healthy diet along with a few hours of gym time every week while still young, you're sure to reap the benefits once the years start passing you by.

With all these physical benefits and more, it's easy to get motivated to start an exercise routine right away. For us ladies with ADHD, it's important to remember that you need to start slow in order to avoid feeling demotivated within the first week or two.

You want to create a routine that lasts, and you want to stay as excited about it tomorrow as you are today. You can set goals for yourself in order to keep yourself motivated. They don't have to be weight-related. They could be as simple as running an extra mile every week or lifting an extra set of weights in two weeks.

Mental Health and More

Now that we've taken a look at some of the physical benefits, let's head on over to the mental health benefits. Firstly, exercise promotes the release of dopamine, which mimics what a lot of medication prescribed especially for ADHD is meant to do. For this reason, many doctors might recommend exercise along with medications, or even as an alternative to medication, depending on the severity of your symptoms.

Exercise has been proven to reduce stress and anxiety in most people. This is crucial for people who have ADHD, as stress and anxiety tend to be magnified in us. It is also said to increase levels of the brain-derived neurotrophic factor, which is a protein involved in learning and memory (Watson, 2012). This protein isn't particularly in high supply for people with ADHD.

Some other benefits are that regular exercise will also help you to improve your memory and it might even reduce impulsive behavior by improving impulse control (Watson, 2012).

To further reduce the risk of becoming demotivated or bored with your workout routine, you should try to engage in varied workouts during the week. Try to chop and change your routine as much as possible. You could even attend a few classes at your local gym, such as yoga or pilates, as these exercises are not only good for your health but your spiritual well-being as well.

Here Are Some Fun Exercises That You Can Try:

- Jogging
- Brisk walking
- Swimming
- Biking
- Sports
- Dancing
- Yoga
- Pilates
- Spinning classes

Anything that gets your heart pumping generates a sweat, and anything that generates a sweat is considered to be an exercise. That means that you can try anything that you enjoy! There is no specific exercise that will help manage your symptoms of ADHD more or less.

While there are certain exercises that benefit different areas of your body, most exercises are good for your mental health, as long as you remember to not overdo it. It might be a fun activity for the whole family if you could participate in sports together or play certain sports such as soccer, basketball, or tennis together.

Calming Techniques

Calming techniques have long been thought to also help you improve your focus and overall concentration. So, along with helping you to calm yourself or to stop a panic attack in its tracks, it might also help you to further train your brain.

The first well-known tip that we've all heard of before is simply breathing. There are breathing techniques that can help stabilize your emotions along with shifting your focus from whatever has been making you feel anxious toward your breathing.

Some people have suggested that you take long and deep breaths, in through the nose and out through the mouth. You can repeat this as many times as you feel is necessary. It's not only for anxious or stressful situations, you can also practice your breathing when you're calm. The trick is to actually focus (yes, focus) on your breathing without getting distracted.

Another tip that I've come across is called 'positive visualization.' By focusing on what you want to achieve and how calm and concentrated you want to be, you might actually achieve it. See yourself as the successful woman that you know you can be; see yourself as calm and collected. This can help you escape a moment of panic as well as get your head on the right track for improvement of concentration.

This next one might sound funny, but it works. It's been suggested that saying your ABCs backward can reduce stress and anxiety. Do you know what else it does? Forces you to concentrate. Nobody knows the ABCs backward by heart. This means that your concentration will be put to the test, and the more you do it, the more you'll remember it and the easier it'll become. That means that it'll also help your memory!

Chapter 6:

Interesting Facts About the History of ADHD

While researching ADHD and how I could cope with the condition (which ultimately led me to write this book), I began wondering about the history. I thought about how difficult life must have been for individuals who might not have known about their condition. Imagine life with such an altering condition, with no way of understanding it or treating it.

This led me to a different kind of research in order to answer different kinds of questions. You must have wondered at some point, too. That's why I decided to add this chapter! Hopefully, this will answer any questions that you may have about the past.

Where It All Began

In 1798, a condition was described by a Scottish doctor that involved symptoms similar to what we know as ADHD today. Sir Alexander Crichton first noticed the lack of concentration in his patients that led him to believe that it was a real condition and not just a random occurrence. He also noticed that it began early in life.

Sir George Frederic Still was a British pediatrician. He first mentioned "an abnormal defect of moral control in children" in 1902 (Holland, 2015). His findings were that affected children seemed to have trouble with controlling their behavior but that they were considered intelligent. This is where the real history starts, as we are unsure about the happenings of 1798.

For the next 35 years, treatment varied considerably. Most experts of the time didn't really know what to make of the condition. In 1922, Alfred. F Tredgold suggested that the symptoms were psychological and not simply bad behavior. And in 1923, Franklin Ebaugh suggested that ADHD could result from brain injury as well.

There was a breakthrough in 1936 when the CDC approved a stimulant medicine called Benzedrine. It was in 1937 that Charles Bradley realized that the medicine helped many children to behave more appropriately.

He also noticed that the medication seemed to help them keep their concentration for a little longer. Unfortunately, his findings were not taken seriously for years. Methylphenidate was first made in 1944, but it didn't receive its official name until 1954: Ritalin. This medication is still used for treatment to this day in both children and adults.

As you might imagine, the first years of research and medication largely excluded young girls and women. The first symptoms related more to boys disrupting classrooms than they did to girls with internal struggles. The girls who did have disruptive behavior were few in numbers. Actually, when you look even further down history, you'll see that mental health wasn't taken very seriously in women at all.

Women were diagnosed with "hysteria," but that was about as scientific as you'd think it to be. Treatment was also seriously lacking. Although hysteria did lead to the first vibrators as a form of treatment. So, there's that.

Ritalin was actually developed to treat chronic fatigue and even depression. Luckily, there was a bit of an understanding of depression during the early 1900s, where it was previously not very well researched. Experts found that Ritalin worked best in treating ADHD, or at least some of its symptoms.

Another interesting fact is that ADHD wasn't actually recognized as a mental disorder until later. In 1952, the very first Diagnostic and Statistical Manual of Mental Disorders (DSM) was issued. The first manual did not include the condition; however, the second edition in 1968 did include it.

From 1970 onwards, there was growing concern about stimulant drug abuse. Most of the drugs that were prescribed to treat ADHD and other conditions were highly addictive and dangerous when not used as directed by a healthcare practitioner. For this reason, there was a law passed in 1970 that limited the amount of time that a person could use these kinds of drugs and how many refills they could get. This helped the situation somewhat, but more dangerous versions of stimulant drugs have since surfaced. As we all know, illicit drugs are, unfortunately, all over today.

The condition was called "hyperkinetic reaction of childhood" at first, but this was changed to "attention deficit disorder" in 1980. Today, it's been changed once again to the name we know: "attention deficit hyperactivity disorder."

With the third and fourth editions of the manual, the information on this condition has been growing rapidly. More and more diagnoses are being made daily. It's probably safe to say that we can thank our stars that we live in this age. But who knows? Perhaps in the future, the experts might look back at our treatment options and think them old-fashioned or even barbaric.

What the Future May Hold

Even in our enlightened age, there is still a lot of research to be conducted. Experts have been working day in and day out to provide us with all the information that we have today. There are thousands of research studies and papers being published. By 2017, there were over 31,000 (Harrar, 2016).

Combining Medication

Brain scans revealed that combining certain medications offered more benefits. In a study by The University of California Los Angeles, 208 children and teenagers were given guanfacine medications such as Intuniv and Tenex, or they were given d-methylphenidate medications such as Ritalin and Concerta. Some of them were given a combination of the two (Harrar, 2016). The study lasted about eight weeks.

The findings were conclusive. A combination of medications seemed to improve ADHD symptoms significantly (Harrar, 2016). Of course, treatment such as this has risks as well. Overuse of stimulants can negatively impact your health, and the combination treatment may even cause a higher risk of dehydration. Further research will be necessary.

Other New Treatments

More and more people are shying away from medication. As an adult, you might feel the same way. Women are particularly prone to negative side effects from certain medications. This isn't medically backed, but simply an observation. Whatever your reason may be, you'll be happy to hear that there are more and more treatments on the rise that don't require any medicines.

As mentioned before, your doctor will know which treatments will work best for you, so taking their advice might be in your best interest. That's just my two cents, and it still remains a personal choice.

Researchers and doctors are working around the clock to develop new treatments and medications. When you look at where humanity began, from thinking that mental health disorders were caused by demonic possession… to a complex understanding of the brain and the chemicals that it releases, it's hard to believe that we've come so far.

In less than two hundred years, we've learned more about mental and physical health than all of humanity has in thousands of years. This is because technology is rapidly advancing, and this means that our experts have more resources for their research.

Perhaps the future might be even brighter for future generations. There might come a day when mental health disorders are a thing of the past. For now, we use what we have to improve our lives and hope that we get to see what amazing things will be discovered or created next!

Chapter 7:

The Positive Side of ADHD

(Surprising Strengths)

We've covered almost every negative aspect of ADHD, from lingering symptoms to treatments and everything in between. It might be time to look at the situation from a different perspective. There have been reports of people with ADHD who have "superpowers." Okay, I don't mean laser vision or the ability to breathe under water, I'm talking about realistic superpowers.

People often forget that there are surprising strengths that can come with the condition; there is so much negativity surrounding ADHD that many don't even realize the talents or abilities that we might have, or that they might have themselves!

Superpowers

As a child, I didn't realize that I was different. I noticed how much extra trouble I was getting into in class for not paying attention and my friends often teased me for "zoning out." But, that was it. It wasn't until I started participating in group projects and started going to playdates that I realized the true extent.

My teachers were in awe of my problem-solving skills, and I was shocked at how different playtime was for other children. It's different for every person; some people with ADHD have a little trouble with problem-solving, others are masters at it. There's something about the way our thoughts jump all over the place that makes it easier for us to see unique solutions that neurotypical people might miss.

When it came to playing, I guess you could have called me a strange kid. I had the wildest imagination, and anything could be a toy, even a piece of grass! I was shocked to learn that other children didn't see the world the way I did. Yes, I was teased for this, too.

The point is, to this day, I am blessed with these skills. My problem-solving skills have gotten me out of many disasters, and my wild imagination led to incredible creativity! It has been said that most people with ADHD are creative and imaginative people. "People with ADHD don't think outside of the box; we create our own fortresses with our unbounded imagination and creativity" (ADDitude Editors, 2016).

Something else that I've noticed and read about is extreme compassion. People with ADHD, especially women, tend to be more compassionate toward each other and others. It's believed that being different makes us see the struggles that other people might face. Even if they're nothing like the ones we face, tender compassion still exists for those who struggle.

In a way, I see this in myself, too. I always root for the player or actor who seems to come from an unfortunate background or who has more obstacles to overcome to succeed than most. I don't really care for the term, but I suppose we could say "the underdog."

It has also been observed that people with ADHD have curious minds, and our brains seem to be wired in a way that makes new concepts and adventures very intriguing. Of course, as with any talent, this does not relate to every individual. But for those of you who have noticed this in yourselves or a loved one, you understand.

With a curious mind often comes an exceptional ability to observe and perceive. People with ADHD often wonder about what could be, instead of looking only at what is now. This skill comes in handy throughout your childhood and adult life.

If you're hungry for adventure and new things, you're likely to not let the fear of change or the "what if" concept keep you from going after personal or occupational goals. The way we see the world is often described as a "bird's eye view" (ADHD Superpowers, 2020)

Some children with ADHD prefer a different kind of learning which involves more hands-on activity and visual stimulation. In adulthood, this can be developed into incredible skills that may seem hard to believe to other people. These skills can include hands-on types of work in which the person with ADHD might excel beyond expectation. They can also include artistic talents and different perspectives.

Have you ever heard of hyperfocus? Hyperfocus is when an individual with ADHD goes into a different kind of state. Instead of a lack of concentration, the individual goes into, well, hyperfocus. This often happens with jobs or projects that the person truly enjoys or has an interest in. These episodes lead to immense productivity and they deliver high-quality outcomes.

Some people with ADHD are naturally flexible and intelligent, along with other mentioned superpowers that lead to great leadership skills. The role of a leader is not simply to lead but to guide. In order to do that, there needs to be compassion, strength, intelligence, curiosity, adaptability, and the ability to speak their mind when others would rather stay silent. Of course, as a leader, one would understand the importance of kindness and constructive criticism. These are all qualities that have been observed in people with ADHD.

The qualities that we might not possess can be learned and perfected. The ones that we've always had should be nurtured and developed. I believe that this begins in childhood. If you can see that a child is creative and curious but has no interest in math, then develop their skills! Sure, we all need basic math in our adult lives, but this is just an example.

If our specific skills are not dampened as kids, just imagine how amazingly bright we'd shine as adults. The school system won't likely be changing any time soon, but as parents of family members, we can help our kids develop in ways that were not granted to us as kids. Be the adult that you needed as a kid!

Super Women

Interesting unrelated fact: a lot of the women we look up to today had/have ADHD!

Lisa Ling

Lisa Ling is a successful and well-known journalist who has worked with *National Geographic*, among other publications. She also has a docuseries called "Our America with Lisa Ling." According to Ling, she was researching ADHD for an article when she started relating to the symptoms more and more.

Ling was diagnosed with ADHD at the age of 40, when she explained a sense of relief. She finally knew what she had been battling against all her life. She finally had a name for it, and more importantly, she had treatment options.

Emma Watson

Watson is a successful actress known for her role as Hermoine Granger in the Harry Potter films. She has allegedly never spoken about her condition, but it is known that she has been receiving treatment for ADHD since childhood.

She's a great example of how manageable ADHD can be when it's diagnosed and treated early.

Simone Biles

Simone Biles is probably the most well-known American gymnast. Her success has been achieved through incredibly hard work and endurance. She often talks about her ADHD on social media, and she's not ashamed to admit that she's on medication.

Here's a young woman who is happy and thriving. Thanks to treatment and the support of her loved ones, she's never let her condition get in the way of her dreams and goals.

Mary-Kate Olsen

We've all heard the name, as the Olsen twins grew up with a lot of us. From television series to movies and books, they've been the stars for years. Today, they're more inclined to fashion than they are to acting. Their success has been magnificent to witness and inspiring to many young women.

What a lot of people don't know is that Mary-Kate Olsen actually has ADHD. Mary-Kate was diagnosed with ADHD as a child and has spent her whole life living with and treating her condition. She never once let it get in her way, and she was very lucky to have the people around her support her as much as they did. She has even stated that she was given more time to finish her exams during her university years in New York. She admits that it takes her longer to register certain things than it takes other people (Castañeda, 2016).

Margaux Joffe

Joffe is an award-winning producer who is also known for being the spearheader for Verizon Media Accessibility and Inclusion. She was diagnosed as an adult at the age of 29, and she explains that she couldn't find a lot of information online for women such as herself and therefore founded Kaleidoscope Society, which is an online community for women with ADHD (Park, 2019).

Her dedication towards the cause has inspired many women around the world, and her passion for women who have the same condition as her sparks union among these women. It's easy to see through Margaux Joffe what a difference you can make.

Women suffering from ADHD are warriors. They fight for their symptoms to be investigated, diagnosed, and treated. Then they battle to thrive in a male-dominated society; and these seven prominent girls demonstrate that they can occasionally win big! They embraced themselves with their ADHD and achieved greatness!

Roxy Olin

Roxy Olin's parents called her "Rollover" because she performed somersaults all around the house all the time. "I stood out because my brother was so calm and orderly," Olin, who has been on MTV's *The City and The Hills*, adds.

"When I was little, my parents sensed that something was wrong with me," she explains. "I struggled in school and was often in trouble. I recall studying for a big test in third grade. I knew all of my vocabulary words by heart, but I only got one right since a student had harmed himself and needed sutures. When I took the test, I was so preoccupied that I couldn't recall anything."

Olin went to the doctor and had been given Ritalin, which she did not like. Her parents and she tried to handle her ADHD without medication until she was properly diagnosed as a teen and put on Adderall.

She crumbled when she attended a drug recovery program that didn't allow her to use her ADHD medication. In two months, she was involved in five car accidents. Many of her friends felt that adult ADHD did not exist.

"My therapist spoke up for me, informing the rehab directors that I required Adderall." "On top of that, he informed them that adult ADHD exists because he has it," Olin adds. "Eventually, he taught me the organizational and time-management techniques that helped him excel in his work."

Olin uses these and other tactics to stay on track in her prominent post. "If I receive a call at 11:30, I write at 10:30." When she's on set rehearsing, she uses her ADHD to give her characters more depth.

Her connections are hampered by ADHD. "When I'm out with someone, I'll tell them about my ADHD. If the individual does not understand or becomes frustrated, he or she shouldn't be around me. At this stage in my life, I've realized that this is a part of who I am. You are not required to conceal your ADHD."

Robin Stephens

Being a professional organizer and having ADHD appear to be an unlikely combination. But it makes sense to Robin Stephens. Before her illness, she ran Your Life in Order, a firm that helped clients achieve order in their homes and lives.

"You are drawn to what you reflect," says Stephens, a behavioral psychology graduate of the University of Washington. "I couldn't operate or focus in a crowded setting."

Stephens, as a girl, didn't quite understand why she couldn't remain still in class. She also was a perfectionist; she could not even start a new project until the previous one was finished. Stephens discovered she had bipolar illness as an adult. She eventually found the connection between bipolar illness and ADHD. Stephens chose to get tested for the illness after struggling to focus on her new profession as a health coach for several years.

"It was complete and utter relief," she recalls. "I feel that if you know what you're dealing with, you can cope with it."

Stephens has techniques and tactics to assist her to control her symptoms as a result of her work with others who have ADHD. She couldn't go a day without making to-do lists, breaking major chores down into digestible portions, and scheduling regular breaks. Two helpers assist her in staying organized.

Stephens has unlimited energy and speaks at breakneck speed, and she often wonders where her personality ends and ADHD starts. Her personality has an impact on her dating life. It has frightened some males. "Some individuals just can't handle it," she adds. "However, after all this time, I've realized it has to be okay to be myself."

Evelyn Polk-Green

"I can multitask because of ADHD," Evelyn Polk-Green explains. "It helps me keep track of all of my work."

Polk-Green, a past president of ADDA and a program director at Illinois STAR Net, an organization that gives education to parents and educators, understands directly that having ADHD has advantages. Her purpose is to help the rest of the world comprehend them.

Polk-Green excelled in a disciplined educational setting throughout elementary and high school; however, as a freshman at Duke University, she struggled to manage her days. She departed without completing her education. She married and gave birth to a kid. She returned to school, despite having an infant at home and a full-time job, and earned her bachelor's and master's degrees in early childhood education from National-Louis University in Chicago.

Polk-Green didn't realize she was living with ADHD until her oldest kid was diagnosed with the disease at the age of seven. "I read a lot about it," she explains. "I said to myself, 'Oh my God, that's me.'"

She finally realized why she could be great at work, handling many tasks at once and hyper-focusing on commitments, but just couldn't keep her home in order. Although she was able to function without medicine for many years, she now believes that it is essential. "It's the difference between being frustrated and productive."

Her words of wisdom for other women? "Determine how the disease impacts you," she advises. "Then, to overcome your deficiencies, employ your strengths." This may imply requesting assistance when necessary. "Decide on a plan, whether it's medicine, treatment, or hiring a cleaner, and stick to it." Your life will improve.

Katherine Ellison

Katherine Ellison was always clear about what she intended to do with her life. She wrote her first magazine piece when she was 11 years old, which sparked an interest in writing and set her on the path to becoming a writer.

Ellison found it difficult to focus in school at times, but writing helped her. "Writing saved me," she adds.

Ellison worked as a foreign reporter for the *San Jose Mercury News* after graduating from Stanford University with a degree in communications and international affairs. The fast-paced environment of the newsroom complemented her abilities. Her work, however, was inconsistent: a Pulitzer Prize at the age of 27 was tainted by inaccuracies in several of her articles.

Ellison sought help from a therapist because she couldn't understand her inconsistencies. She had the impression that she was undermining her efforts. Ellison didn't realize she had ADHD until she was 49, when her oldest kid was diagnosed.

Ellison understood her employment issues were caused by ADHD. She has attempted a variety of treatments to control her ADHD symptoms, including metacognition, meditation, neurofeedback, exercise, and sometimes medication. These, combined with tons of forgiveness, have been the most beneficial to her.

It was difficult for Ellison to listen to family and friends in the past, but she is now more mindful of how she behaves around people. She tries hard to keep the connections in her life intact. Her book *Buzz: A Year of Paying Attention* details Ellison's attempts to bond with her kid even though they both have ADHD. "Acknowledging my ADD and becoming more calm has helped me be less reactive to my son," she adds.

Finding one's passion, according to Ellison, is essential for navigating life with ADHD. "I picked a task that was ideal for the way my brain functions."

Cynthia Gerdes

Cynthia Gerdes, an entrepreneur, sees ADHD as a benefit. "It's simple to accomplish a million things at once," she explains.

Gerdes began her teaching career before becoming the owner of Hell's Kitchen, an award-winning restaurant in Minneapolis that pulls in more than a million dollars each year. Before going into the restaurant industry, she operated numerous successful toy businesses. Gerdes, who has bachelor's degrees in teaching and business management from the University of North Carolina, was always able to work the long hours her employment required, but she struggled with simple things like grocery shopping.

"I couldn't cook," she confesses. "I couldn't acquire the five components I required even with a supermarket list."

Gerdes went to see her doctor, who handed her a form to fill out more about her symptoms. She finally realized why she had more energy than anyone else when she discovered she had ADHD.

Gerdes blames ADHD for some of her conduct, particularly her repeated professional changes. She feels that the illness enables her to get a project started but forces her to move on once things settle into a pattern. This is why Gerdes opened a restaurant once her toy businesses became established.

The restaurant executive discovered that adjusting her routine would be enough to keep her ADHD under control. "I won't do two meetings in a row because I know I can't sit still for that long," she adds. Taking pauses while studying menus and invoices is also beneficial.

She is still having difficulties with food shopping. Her spouse, a chef, is encouraging. "When I spin in circles around the home, he is both delighted and puzzled," she adds. "Thank goodness he's a cook!"

Patricia Quinn

"I'm not the type of person who believes ADHD is a strength, but I do think you can use it to become successful," says Dr. Patricia Quinn, a Washington, D.C.-based psychologist.

Quinn wasn't hyper as a youngster, although she did have periods of intensity. She didn't hear her mother shouting to her from another room, but she was able to concentrate on her studies for hours. "I was impulsive as well," she admits. "I threw myself into everything and, happily, succeeded."

Quinn picked medicine as a profession because it was tough. However, she had difficulties while entering medical school at Georgetown University. Quinn could recall and understand what was said in lectures, but she struggled to retain knowledge from textbooks. She sought therapy, but no one recognized adults might have ADHD at the time.

Quinn focused on early childhood development and began conducting ADHD studies. She discovered in 1972 that the attributes that had helped her succeed in medical school—impulsivity and hyperactivity—were symptoms of the disease.

Quinn's current purpose is to raise awareness of the issues that women and girls with ADHD face. She co-founded The National Center for Girls and Women with ADHD in 1997 with Kathleen Nadeau, Ph.D., and she has published numerous publications on the subject. She feels that the illness frequently stays misdiagnosed in girls and women since it does not produce hyperactivity in men. "Because girls and women don't annoy anyone, they don't even get diagnosed."

Quinn, who hasn't used medication to control her symptoms, says finding she had the disease helped her understand why she felt so unique from other medical students. She feels that, in the end, it was a hard effort that led her to where she is now. "Despite my ADHD, I achieved a lot of success," she adds.

Sari Solden

Sari Solden is in the stigmatizing impact of ADHD. Years ago, after finishing a meal at a social gathering, ladies were supposed to get up, bring their dishes through into the kitchen, and put everything back where they belonged. "It's like a dance after the dinner," Solden explains. "Me? All I did was stand there, frozen."

Such experiences have affected Solden's career and life, since she focuses on the effects of ADHD on women. She knows the embarrassment many women with ADD feel when they are unable to organize things, stay ahead of the family routine, maintain friendships, or keep their homes immaculate.

Solden began her job in a big family assistance agency after receiving a master's degree in clinical counseling from California State University. She struggled with administrative tasks and focused on extensive customer lists. To assist her focus, she frequently turned off clocks and fans inside the office.

Solden began to learn further about adults and learning impairments via her employment, and she recognized her symptoms like attention deficit. Solden was relieved when she heard the word "ADHD" from a doctor. "It was emancipating," she adds.

Solden is now in private practice and has learned to arrange her work and personal lives. She outlines the obstacles that women with ADHD experience in her book Women with Attention Deficit Disorder and provides techniques for negotiating society's expectations. "Women with ADHD must recognize that their brains function differently," she adds, "and not blame themselves."

Solden claims that meeting fellow women with ADHD has aided her since they understand how her mind functions. "I learn from the ladies with ADHD with whom I work. They empower me."

These are only a few. There are thousands of them out there! You can be one of them, too! Don't let your ADHD be an excuse to fail, let it be your reason for striving toward greatness! Especially if you might be the mother of young children who may also have been diagnosed with this condition; be the example that you wish you had when you were younger and confused about what was happening to you. Knowing that all these inspirational superheroes encourage women with ADHD really feels empowering. You can be a heroine just like them and take pride in yourself even with ADHD!

Chapter 8:

Debunking Myths About ADHD

There are many common misconceptions about ADHD, so many that they are hard to miss. You've probably heard some of them either as a child or as an adult. They might have been spat at you by people who were trying to be hurtful or they might simply have been out of misinformation. Either way, these need to be debunked so we can set the record straight!

The Most Common Myths

1. The first myth that we've already tackled is the myth that boys are more likely to have ADHD than girls. Throughout this book, we've basically already debunked this one. You know now that this is a misconception that stemmed from a lack of research and information.

2. This might be hard to believe for some, since ADHD has been a recognized medical condition for a while now, as mentioned before. There are actually people who still believe that ADHD is not a real medical condition. You read that right, even in this age of enlightenment, there are still those who simply don't "believe." This has been proven by more than just brain scans and research.

3. This third one is probably something that some of you could have heard from someone who was trying to be malicious or ignorant. Another common myth is that people who have ADHD are lazy and need to try harder. As we've discussed, this is not the case. There are logical reasons for procrastination and

it takes a whole lot more than simply "trying" to overcome other symptoms of ADHD.

4. This was also previously covered, but I thought I'd mention it again. It's not true that people who have ADHD can't *ever* focus; as we now know, hyperfocus is real! And it can be intense when it occurs. Some people have these episodes frequently, others have them infrequently or not at all. It all depends on the individual.

5. You want to know what really grinds my gears? The same people who don't "believe" in ADHD actually believe that children who have ADHD are simply misbehaving. "They need discipline." Yeah, since we know how serious ADHD is and how it affects a person's life, I think it's safe to say that this myth can be laid to rest.

6. ADHD can sometimes make learning new things difficult when undiagnosed and untreated; unfortunately, this has led to the myth that ADHD is a learning disability. Let's bury this one, too. ADHD is not a learning disability, although it can exist along with actual learning disabilities.

7. This next one is pretty hurtful, and I can imagine that it must have a very negative effect on the parents who've heard it. There is a common myth that ADHD is caused by bad parenting. This, like most of the other myths, comes from ignorance and misinformation.

8. As we know from first-hand experience and information provided in this book, children don't outgrow ADHD. So it goes without saying that this is another myth that we get to bury.

9. Now, there are some people who think that ADHD medications are similar to certain illicit drugs and that taking them will make a person seem as if they have been taking these illicit drugs and are equally as dangerous. This is completely false; the only similarity between some ADHD medications and

these illicit drugs is that both are stimulants. Coffee is also a stimulant, so... The truth is that if medications have been prescribed and they are taken in the recommended doses, then they are completely safe. All medications have adverse effects if taken differently from the prescribed dose, and a lot of other common medications can also be addictive if not controlled.

10. There seems to be concern about whether psychostimulants are still effective after puberty. Let me assure you that they are. Adults and teenagers who use these medications continue to benefit from them.

Why It's Important to Spread Awareness

With so many misconceptions and so much misinformation, it's important to spread awareness in order to correct these myths. Misinformation such as this can lead to shame and guilt, which may keep the affected people from proper diagnosis and treatment.

The stigma that surrounds ADHD is toxic, at best, and it may contribute to the ongoing suffering of people around the world who have this condition either knowingly or unknowingly.

ADHD is one of the most common mental conditions in children. In children who aren't diagnosed, chaos can erupt in their lives and the lives of the people in whose care they are.

It's not something that we want to know, but there are children and adults who get bullied and treated differently for being, well, different. In a perfect world, this wouldn't be an issue, but we live in an imperfect world. Therefore, it's our duty to spread awareness in order to ease the suffering of ourselves and others!

What You Can Do to Help

The best way to spread information is by speaking out. Many people have no experience with ADHD and therefore don't know any better than what they've heard from others. Therefore, it's a good way to help by telling people about your own experiences or those of your loved ones.

ADHD Awareness Month falls in October, and this is a great time to take part in activities that aid the spread of information. You can search the internet for events and other ways in which you can get involved. There are many organizations that take part in ADHD Awareness Month such as CHADD.

You also don't have to wait for the designated month. You can spread awareness every day. Social media has become a powerful tool for this very reason. You can make updates on your situation or simply share a few educational articles now and then. It really doesn't matter how you choose to do it, as long as you do commit to doing it.

It's not only for your own sake but for the sake of everyone out there who lives under constant scrutiny and judgment. With the right amount of love and respect, we can help so many people!

Chapter 9:

Self-Care

We've spoken about the importance of self-care. Sleep is probably the most important form of self-care that there is, and we know that by now. But as a woman who has ADHD, you need to shift the focus onto yourself more often than most. Your world is already so difficult and full of constant struggling. Taking care of yourself is important for both you and your family members.

The more rested, calm, and taken care of you are, the better you can function. In order for you to be the best mom, wife, friend, or employee that you can be, you need to make your health a priority. Self-care relates to both your physical health and your mental health.

Self-Care Ideas

Know Your Limits

People with ADHD often have to deal with more than they're comfortable with. Life forces us into new situations all the time, and that's great. As mentioned before, some of us thrive on new experiences and adventures, but some of us don't. That's okay, you need to focus on your limitations just as much as you focus on pushing yourself.

Self-care is also about knowing when you need to stop or take a break, at the very least. There is no shame in admitting that you have limits, everyone does. Knowing your limits will help ensure that you don't reach burnout status. Burnout can be demotivating and upsetting but can be avoided if you pay attention to your mind and body.

Meditation

Meditation is probably one of the most popular forms of self-care. There are various forms of meditation. You're bound to find one that works for you. Meditation helps improve your concentration, too, and it also relieves stress and anxiety, which we know is abundant for a lot of us.

Facials, Nail Care, Massages

This is probably my favorite form of self-care. Who doesn't like getting pampered? Turns out, it's pretty good for your mental health. Just like most forms of self-care, these pamperings relieve stress and anxiety. They may even relieve symptoms of depression, but this has not been scientifically proven.

FOOD AND WINE!

Okay, most doctors would probably not agree with this statement. But I believe that the *occasional* indulgence is good for you! Stressing on the word *occasional* because there is a fine line between what's good for you and what can turn into a bad habit that diminishes your health.

To me, there's nothing quite as relaxing as having a glass of wine with a good meal and my significant other. Whatever works, right?

Take a Walk

Vitamin D is crucial for your health, and your body doesn't make it on its own. The sun is our primary source of Vitamin D. If you're not getting enough Vitamin D, this can lead to symptoms of depression; therefore, it's a good idea to get out and breathe in a bit of fresh air every now and again!

Wash Wash Wash!

Many years ago, it was thought to be healing to wash yourself or to take their variation of a bath. Today, we know that while taking a bath might not cure your disease, it will help you feel better.

Dress to Impress… Yourself!

Even when you're just at home, you can still feel good about yourself. If you feel beautiful and comfortable in flip-flops, that's fine. But if you're like me and you enjoy getting all dressed up, go for it!

It's not for anyone else but yourself. A friend of my mother's used to say that she always felt better after putting her makeup on and wearing something nice, even when she was sick. Can looking nice cure your illness? Probably not, but at least you'll feel pretty.

Try Going Without Electronics

You should try to get as much time away from your electronics as you can. Your eyes need the rest, and so does your brain! Self-care is also about conserving the mental energy that it requires to spend time on your cellphone or laptop.

Loved ones need to understand that you need this time to yourself. You can politely explain to anyone who might want to reach you that you're not switching your phone off to be rude but simply to give yourself a mental break.

Spend Time With People You love

Sometimes, some alone time can be crucial to our sanity, but so can family time. As a mother, I often find comfort in the little hugs and kisses that my children offer. These little creatures don't always realize that while I may be the one keeping them alive, they're the ones who are keeping me from derailing.

From the perspective of a woman who doesn't have or want children, I can understand how this may sound a little silly. It's okay to not want or even like children. Your life and future are in your hands. In this day and age, you get to choose whether you want to be a mother or not. And if you do choose not to have children, then plant babies or fur babies count, too!

Whether it's your family, friends, kids, significant other, pets, or plants, the sense of comfort will be the same. You know that you're not alone, but it can be helpful and comforting to have that bit of reassurance.

Toxic Self-Care

There is a common misconception that self-care is overindulging in alcohol and changing your hair or even having multiple partners. Please, don't fall into this type of thinking. If there is one thing that you need to remember then it's this: self-care means taking care of your mental and physical self by engaging in healthy habits or exercises that benefit you in both regards.

Toxic self-care is real, and the internet seems to be full of it these days. Do whatever makes you happy as long as it's not harmful to you or anyone around you. Do whatever makes you happy as long as it doesn't end up making things worse.

Remember that many bad habits result in certain positive feelings for a fleeting moment, but these never last, and you might end up feeling even worse after.

Chapter 10:

Embrace Who You Are, Accept Yourself

Throughout your life, you may have felt out of place or as if you just couldn't be what everyone expected you to be. I often read about women who live with a constant sense of self-resentment, and the phrases "I wish I was normal" or "I wish I was somebody else" come up frequently. This truly breaks my heart. To have these kinds of feelings about yourself is difficult to deal with, especially when it's on a daily basis. Always be confident in who you are.

Confidence makes us feel prepared for the challenges of life. When we are confident, we are more inclined to pursue opportunities and chances rather than shy away from them. And if things aren't working out the first time, confidence encourages us to try again.

When confidence is low, the reverse occurs. People who lack confidence may be less likely to try new things or meet new people. If they fail the first time, they may be less likely to attempt again. People who lack confidence may be unable to realize their full potential.

In these moments, I wish I could simply reach out and offer a reassuring hug or some other form of comfort. Some would say that you might not be normal, but you're perfectly abnormal. And that makes you beautiful! What's so great about being "normal" anyway? Even as we joke about this, I know that it's a sore subject for some. In reality, you are completely normal. Just a different variation of normal. "What's normal for the spider is chaos for the fly."

Newly Diagnosed as an Adult Woman

As we move further along this journey, it's important to reach out to the older women who might have recently been diagnosed. Your whole life is about to change, and that's a big deal. You could be feeling relieved as your difficult life suddenly makes sense. You might be feeling anxious because of impending treatments or you might even be feeling somewhat depressed after spending your life thinking that you were one person but realizing that you might be another person. This isn't accurate, though. You're still the same woman that you were yesterday; the only difference is that you now know how to improve your quality of life!

It's long been thought that while adults don't outgrow ADHD, they do outgrow most of the hyperactivity, which, as you know, can then manifest as impulsivity. From my experience, this isn't *always* the case. I've come across very hyperactive women who, for example, have an inability to sit still for long periods of time. The energy from these women can often be described as nothing short of explosive. To be honest, it's quite pleasant to be in their company. But I can imagine that it can't always be as pleasant for the woman with the symptoms.

So you've noticed these symptoms in yourself. Whether it's explosive energy or impulsivity, or everything in between, you've gone ahead and reached out for help. Firstly, congratulations! You've taken the first step to a healthier and happier life!

The next few weeks will probably be the hardest. Coming to terms with a diagnosis such as this at an advanced age isn't easy. The most important thing that you can do now is to ensure that you have a support system. You'll need all the love and care from your family and friends, and you're welcome to ask them for a bit of patience during this trying time.

The second most important thing to remember is to stick to your treatment plan. Most ADHD medications can take anywhere from a few days to a week or two to start showing positive effects, and it can take up to two months for the medication to reach its full potential. During this time, you need to remember that whatever you're feeling right now is only temporary.

It is during this time when many women make the biggest mistake: they abandon treatment for fear of ineffectiveness. It takes time for these things to work, and it can take even longer for you to get used to your new routine and the new mental space that you might find yourself in.

In order for you to keep yourself on schedule, you can set reminders for when to take your medication and remember to never skip a dose. If you do skip a dose, then it's important to remember that you should never take a double dose to make up for it. Ask your doctor for advice on this matter if you're unsure.

What You May Be Prescribed

There are a few different kinds of medications that are used to treat ADHD in children and adults. By now, you've heard of some of them, such as stimulants and non-stimulants.

Here are a few brand names that you might come across as sourced from an article by Larry Silver, published on December 1st, 2021 in ADDitude (Silver, 2011).

- Adderall XR (amphetamine)
- Concerta (methylphenidate)
- Dexedrine (amphetamine)
- Evekeo (amphetamine)
- Focalin XR (dexmethylphenidate)
- Quillivant XR (methylphenidate)
- Ritalin (methylphenidate)

- Strattera (atomoxetine hydrochloride)

- Vyvanse (lisdexamfetamine dimesylate)

These names may sound a little intimidating, but these medications have been extensively researched and tested to ensure safety and efficacy. If you have any of these on your prescription, don't fear! Trust in your doctor and let them know about any severe side effects, which aren't all that common.

For the first few months, it might be trial and error. Not every medication will work for every person. So, while it's important to give it time to work (as mentioned before), you should still look out for signs that this specific medication might not fit well for you.

If this happens, don't be discouraged! Your ideal treatment is out there and you'll get there.

Just Breathe, You Can Do This

Keep in mind that this is new and completely different. As adults, it can be more difficult to treat ADHD because our patterns have already been set. In children, especially young children, it can be easy to learn new habits or to break old ones because they're still in their formative years. This is a little harder for us. So, don't beat yourself up for not being perfectly capable of every single thing that you're told you need to be able to do just yet.

It takes more time, but that doesn't mean that it's not possible. ADHD can affect our habits, and it can be positive or negative, though I have unfortunately heard of a few more cases of negativity. This simply means that you'll need to acknowledge these bad habits and change them.

ADHD makes social interaction difficult for some. In this case, you might come into the habit of isolating yourself. This is a bad habit! Everyone needs their space, and some of us need a little more than others. But social interaction is still crucial for human beings! We're social creatures by nature and we need each other to thrive; not that you couldn't thrive on your own, but it's more pleasant and easier to do so with the help and support of others.

Fight back and take charge of your life! Once you've accepted the fact that you have ADHD and that it's a part of you, you can then start working on all the other issues that you've now realized might be due to your newly diagnosed condition, such as the one mentioned above.

As you trail through the days that turn into weeks, you might be overcome with an urge to just let go of your emotions and let it all out. Some would suggest that this should be suppressed. I suggest letting it all out. Grab that box of tissues and cry until you feel better. Let it all out and deal with the emotions inside of you. We have a hard enough time dealing with every other aspect of life, don't let your own emotions be your downfall.

Most importantly, you need to be patient with yourself. Everything that you're going through now will eventually be worth it. Small side-effects from medications, jumping emotions, fear, aloof it… once you start seeing results, it'll be worth it and you'll thank yourself.

You Are Worth the Wait

Don't ever feel like you don't deserve help, love, or compassion. You're worthy of all the good things that life has to offer. Every obstacle you've faced has led to this, and every one of them has been a learning experience. Past mistakes don't mean anything, they just mean that you're human.

You'll never feel worthy if you don't accept yourself for the strong and capable woman that you are. Never forget that just because you have a little more trouble with certain things than others, doesn't mean that you aren't just as capable.

Remember what I said about ADHD superpowers? You likely have some of them, too! No matter your age, you're still magnificent to observe in your natural state. You don't need another brain or personality, another body, or even another husband (we love them but some of us have wished this); all you need is your own reassurance.

People won't always be there to offer this, and you might have the best support system in the world and still feel overwhelmed. In this case, your own reassurance will mean more than any other form of support. You need to convince yourself of your worth and capabilities every day. You can repeat positive affirmations to yourself daily. It may sound cheesy, but it works. The more you tell yourself that you are everything that you need to be and that you have everything that you need, the more you'll believe it.

Whatever obstacles you face, the journey is worth the result. Embrace yourself and all the differences that you've previously seen as character flaws. You are so unique! Every simple thing about you proves that, because while there are thousands of people who have ADHD, none of them are you!

Chapter 11:

Decision-Making

Decisions are a part of life regardless of your age or brain development. You'll need to make a million small decisions every day, and a couple of big ones that may impact your life tremendously. Most people have trouble with making big decisions, but when it comes to people with ADHD, even the smallest of choices can sometimes feel like a mountain of disappointment waiting on the other side.

When we do finally make a choice, we're often plagued with regret. Nobody needs this extra stress on their shoulders; making a decision should not be such a traumatic experience.

Tips on How to Take Charge of Your Decisions

Taking charge of your decisions isn't as complicated as it may sound. It just takes a little more thought and dedication to yourself.

Create a Due Date

What may help you as a first step is to give yourself a due date for your decision. Let's say that you need to decide on whether or not to go on a date this weekend. It would be a good idea to make your decision at least two days before the actual date is supposed to take place.

Perhaps you need to decide whether or not you want to take a new job opportunity. This kind of decision should not be taken lightly, and it would be wise to give yourself enough time, if that's at all possible. As long as you know when your decision is due, that should serve as motivation.

The due date doesn't need to be days away, and it depends on the kind of decision that you wish to make. If it's a minor decision and you only have a few hours, then your deadline can be a few minutes away. Don't stress over not having enough time. You're more than capable of making the right choice.

Take the Time to Think

Once you've decided on a deadline, you'll need to take the time to think about the decision that you need to make. This means that you'll need to sit down, clear your mind, and really consider all the possible outcomes.

Weigh the Pros and Cons

With every decision comes two sides; either you do something or you don't. What may help you is to weigh the pros and cons.

Here's an example: The question is life-altering. Do we move to California(for a new job opportunity) or do we stay in New York at the moment?

Pros: A new job, new neighbors, new friends, new experiences, California weather, beautiful beaches, and much more.

Cons: A long trip to see friends and family that will be left behind, missing important family events unless it's possible to travel, etc.

Once you've looked at the decision from all perspectives and you've weighed these, you can go ahead and try to make your decision. For some people, this is enough to help them decide. Write these down and read them out loud to yourself; this can help you fully understand the positive side and the negative side.

Don't Be Afraid to Reach Out to Someone for Help

Some people need a little more than the above in order to make the right decisions, and that's perfectly normal and nothing to be worried about. What may help is speaking to someone you love or care for and trust about the matter. Reading the pros and cons to them will help them understand the situation, and while you shouldn't let someone else make decisions for you, it might help to have someone else give you their opinion.

Their opinion will be from an outside perspective, which could help you see things differently.

No one is designed to do everything on their own. There is no shame in seeking assistance if and when you require it. Begin by consulting with your primary care physician. Explain to them about your specific difficulties or questions, and ask if they have any suggestions for who you should contact or if they recommend you consult a mental health expert. An expert can assist you in reducing distractions and locating methods to increase your attention.

It's also critical to recognize when there are people around you who are eager to assist. Most likely, your friends and family want to help you but are unsure how. Inform the people in your life about your ADHD so that they comprehend your symptoms and treatment, which will enhance your interactions with them.

Whenever it comes to ADHD, social support is essential. It's up to you whom you share things with, but a great place to begin is with your spouse, friends, and close family.

Then you can think about alerting others, such as coworkers, managers, or instructors. ADHD might cause some difficulties at work or school, but the people around you can help you to overcome these hurdles if they understand what you're going through. When you request additional time for a certain assignment, they will be more understanding.

When you've just been diagnosed with a disorder like ADHD, it might be difficult to know how to approach the subject. People might have varying interpretations of what assistance entails, so it's helpful if you can express exactly what you want from them.

Look up ADHD on the internet and compile a list of crucial information to discuss. Depending on what you've studied, compose a phrase or two that defines ADHD in your own words. It may also be beneficial to consider what questions the other individual could ask so that you can prepare appropriate responses.

A support group, in addition to medication and one-on-one counseling, can be a helpful strategy to manage your illness. You can communicate with other individuals with ADHD who understand what you're going through, which helps relieve some of the load on your friends and family.

Support groups are venues where people with ADHD may meet in person or online to share their experiences, knowledge, and coping skills. Local chapters of ADHD organizations, social media, and websites such as Adults and Children with Attention-Deficit/Hyperactivity Disorder (CHADD) or the National Institute of Mental Health might help you discover groups (NIMH).

You could also contact a local social worker, a life coach who works primarily with individuals with ADHD, or a counselor who focuses on cognitive-behavioral treatment for ADHD.

Look Further Than the Here and Now

When faced with decisions that are possibly life-altering, you should always aim to look further than the here and now. You might feel one way now, or be in a certain situation now, but your future may be vastly different. Always consider variables.

The right choice may result in a negative outcome for the short term, but the long-term result will positively impact your life. This is another situation to consider.

Use Your Head!

These days, a lot of people would say that it's wiser to follow your heart, but I'm here to tell you that, while trusting your gut can be a good thing, you need to follow your head in most cases. Especially when it comes to big decisions, you can't let your heart decide where your future will lead if it leads you to failure or heartbreak.

It's important to follow your dreams, but your head needs to always be in control. Think logically about the situation and don't just do what you *think* might make you happy without delving deep into the facts.

What if Your Choice Ends up Being Wrong?

Consider the fact that you might still end up making the wrong choice, even after the most thorough consideration. Even if it isn't the wrong choice, it might still result in a negative outcome.

In this case, you'd need to be prepared to deal with the consequences. Would you be okay if the outcome did blow up? This is not saying that you need to be incredibly negative, as a negative mindset won't get you anywhere. I'm just saying that you need to be prepared.

Be Confident in Your Own Abilities

At least you know that it can only go one of two ways, either wonderfully or it could go wrong. If you're prepared for both, it'll be less devastating if it does go wrong. But until then, be confident in yourself.

If you have made a choice, it is likely because you believed that it would be the best course of action. You're capable of more than you give yourself credit for, and as long as you're sure that you've considered every possible variable, you can rest easy.

Sticking to Your Choices

During the course of your life, you'll make many choices that require commitment and hard work. As a woman with ADHD, you might have trouble sticking to your decisions. We sometimes change our minds too frequently, which can lead to a fusion of negative outcomes.

Stay on Course

So, you've decided to try out a healthier lifestyle by eating right and following a regular exercise plan, or something similar. You went through all the steps and you've made up your mind, but a week or two into this decision, things seem to be getting harder and your motivation starts declining.

This happens to everyone at some point. In this case, it's important to keep your goals in mind in order to stick to the plan. You can motivate yourself by using positive visualizations to see yourself when you've already reached certain goals, and by getting someone to join in on the fun with you! Having a partner or friend to support you can make these kinds of commitments both fun and longer lasting!

The situation might also be minor, such as what to wear or eat. People often don't realize how much pressure and anxiety these simple choices can cause us. And again, how often we change our minds. While these choices may seem insignificant to others, they can be difficult to deal with for us. Some women even prefer that others make these choices for them.

I don't recommend that, again, because you need to be in charge of your life at all times. A choice you make, no matter how small, affects you more than anyone else. For this reason, you need to be the one who decides.

I used to simply close my eyes, stick my hand out while turning one time, and then open my eyes. The thing that I am pointing to is the thing that I choose. Yes, in a few hours I might feel a little regret; what if I had worn the blue dress instead? But that's normal.

Luckily, these little choices don't have too much of an impact on the quality of our lives, but that doesn't mean that they're any less stressful, it just means that whatever we end up choosing won't have catastrophic results. Unless, you know, you choose to wear a bikini to work or eat three-day-old food, then it might result negatively. So uh, don't do that.

Remind Yourself of the Positive Parts

When it comes to the bigger decisions, through whatever hardships you fight, you need to remind yourself of the pros that caused you to make the decision in the first place. Remind yourself about the good things that will come once you've endured the initial stages of difficulty.

Don't give up after a few weeks or let yourself fall into depression simply because things might not be going exactly as expected, yet. If you've prepared yourself for possible failure, you can work through any hiccups that come your way. But even then, keep your eye on the prize.

Avoid Impulsive Decision-Making

For women like us, it can be difficult to consider all these steps and tips for decision-making. I know from personal experience that even if you know what you can do to help you make the right decision, you can still end up making a hasty, impulsive decision.

These can sometimes lead to lifelong consequences. Getting married in Vegas to someone you barely know would be a good example. And so is getting your current partner's name tattooed on you.

Ladies, we struggle with impulsivity, but that doesn't mean that we should simply give in to it and use our condition as an excuse. As grown women with incredible mental capacity, we have the ability to avoid impulsive decisions.

It's not that impulsive decisions are always bad. My grandmother used to decide to go to the beach (an eight-hour drive away) on a whim and then load her entire little bus full of watermelons that she had purchased and spend a day or two selling them for a profit. Off to the beach!

Life is full of adventures, so if you have the means, go for it! The best adventures are the ones we never planned for. But sometimes it's just not worth the risk. Let's say you see a beautiful dress but the price tag is enough to make a celebrity weep. Now, an impulsive decision would be to simply buy it in order to "spoil" yourself.

This can lead to unnecessary financial complications and/or arguments with your significant other. It would be a better idea to assess the situation thoroughly, perhaps you can save up for the dress instead. This might be a simple example, but I'm sure it gets the point across.

Impulsive decisions can also come in different forms, such as interrupting people who are talking or interrupting during meetings. This kind of behavior might not be intentional, and that's why we should focus on them because they can create a negative image of us.

To combat this, you should always wait a few seconds after a new idea has come to mind. Firstly, assess whether the information that you want to share is relevant to the current conversation. Secondly, wait until the person who is currently speaking takes a pause.

It might be difficult to keep your thoughts to yourself. We all have trouble in this regard at one point or another. But it's important that you keep calm and wait. Remember that you will get your turn to speak and that your information will be just as impactful then as it will be now.

Whatever the choice is that you need to make, you can always try and follow these simple steps to ensure that regret is limited and that you don't go changing your mind too often!

Chapter 12:

Managing Your Finances

On top of everything else, we need to manage our finances, too! Impulsive spending can lead to financial damage, as I have mentioned before. But this is not the only thing that we need to manage; there is a lot more to keeping track of your income and outcome than you might think. It can feel overwhelming, but a budget is your best bet.

Keeping track of exactly what you earn and what you spend will help you to save up for that beautiful dress or pair of jeans, or even that vacation! It'll also help you know what kind of financial position you're really in.

This is a short chapter with a little bit of advice gathered from personal experience and a bit of research. Keep in mind that every situation is different.

Budgeting

It doesn't really matter where you document your finances for yourself, as long as it's easily accessible and stored safely. Some people prefer writing this down by hand and others prefer using spreadsheets.

Many people with ADHD dislike looking at their money for one simple fact: It's usually not great news. Even if they know much better cognitively, they choose to assume that all will work out in the end– fingers crossed. The issue is that they have forgotten the first rule of managing money: Money likes attention!

Several persons with ADHD are experts at avoiding direct touch with their money. In a game of financial Russian roulette, they ignore bank statements or let mail pile up for months: "If we don't see the bills, they don't exist, so we don't have to deal with them."

The harsh reality is that tackling your present financial flow—both money that comes in and the money that goes out—is really the only way to regain control. That necessitates an ADHD-friendly budget, as well as these other budgeting suggestions for ADHD minds.

Do whatever works best for you!

1. **Document your income**. Firstly, before taxes and other deductions, and then after these deductions. It's the best idea to work from the income you have left after the necessary deductions have been made.

2. **Create different categories for your spending**. You can label them as groceries, toiletries, utilities, medical bills, rent/mortgage, loans, spending, and so on. Whatever you spend on needs to be documented at this stage.

3. You can **make a list of goals** that you wish to set for yourself. For example, let's say that you want to save $5,000 by the end of the year. You can document these goals in this stage and think about ways you can achieve these goals. Strictly sticking to your budget will mean that it will be easier to achieve your goals because you'll have more control over what goes out. You can put your savings away before budgeting for any spending money or any other non-necessities.

4. **Stick to your budget!** After documenting all of this information, you might need to change a few of your habits in order to reach your goals. This will only affect you positively in the long term, which means that it'll be worth the minor inconveniences that you might need to endure.

5. Remember to **always budget for unexpected situations**. You can't put everything in savings and spend the rest without being

prepared for an unexpected injury or illness. We like to think of ourselves as indestructible, but it's especially important to keep in mind that anything can happen now during a literal global pandemic.

6. It might sound like a lot of work, but you need to **regularly update your budget** and include anything you spend or receive throughout the month. If you can keep track of your budget for at least three months, then this would be enough information to accurately predict when you'll have enough savings for something bigger, such as a house or a car. This can also serve as motivation to keep you going!

These steps might be simple enough for the average person, but they're anything but simple for us! That's why we need to make sure that we actually do the things we plan to do. As always, you can set a daily reminder on your phone with the title "check budget" or something similar. This will help you remember to document daily expenses!

Fixed expenses are expenses such as your rent/mortgage, transport, utilities, etc. Variable expenses are expenses such as food, entertainment, etc. It would be wise to ensure that you understand these terms and under which of these your expenses fall.

Here's an example of a budget that has been set up with these tips in mind.

Income after taxes	$8000
Fixed expenses	
Rent	$2500
Utilities	$500
Gas	$400

Study loan	$500
Savings	$500
Unexpected expenses	$1000
Total	$5400

Unexpected expenses that have not been used by the end of the month could be put toward savings or perhaps toward a family trip. You can even create a separate savings account for unexpected expenses such as medical bills. That way, you won't have to dip into your savings that are meant for a house or university fees, etc.

What's left	**$2600**
Variable expenses	
Food	$1000
Clothes	$200
Internet/Netflix	$300
Nail salon	$100
Hair salon	$250
Other groceries	$500
Spending	$250
Total	$2600

This is a rough and simple example of what your budget can look like. You can add more columns or rows if you want to go into further detail about exactly which groceries you bought or what types of food you bought and what they cost. Here is a small example of what this may look like.

Food	Cost
Meats/protein substitutes	$300
Vegetables	$150
Pasta/rice	$50
Sauces	$50
Milk	$100
Cereals	$100
Coffee	$100
Sugar	$50
Treats	$100
Total	$1000

Let's Talk About Credit Cards

These sneaky little plastic pieces of temptation have a certain way of getting people in trouble. They can be very helpful in certain situations, but the constant temptation can become too much for anyone.

Since some of us have a little trouble with impulsivity, credit cards are probably a hazard that we should avoid. Impulsive spending can lead to debt that can take years to pay off, and this debt can result in severe mental strain that could have been avoided.

When I was younger, I used to say that I wouldn't buy anything if I couldn't buy it in cash. This is, unfortunately, not possible for most people. Life has a way of forcing you into situations that you don't want to be in. Without a great credit score, you can't do anything. This sucks, but it means that credit is necessary.

That doesn't mean that you need to get yourself into so much debt that you can barely keep your head above water. You can put your credit card away somewhere safe so that it doesn't become a temptation every time you go shopping and only take it out when it's absolutely necessary.

You Are Responsible for Your Future

At the end of the day, your finances are your responsibility, and managing them is more important than you think. You don't need a degree in accounting to be able to stay on top of your finances; it's just a little basic budgeting and some self-restraint!

Saving money is vital because it gives stability, release from worry, and independence. And, while there are several reasons to save, you just need to select one that speaks to you. You should prioritize saving, whether it's for helping others, enhancing your household finances, leaving a great financial legacy, or simply having a bit more fun.

Another reason for saving could be for your retirement. You don't want to live on the bare minimum when you retire, you want to be able to travel and live comfortably. Therefore, this is something that you might want to consider when drawing up your budget and deciding on the things you wish to save for.

Chapter 13:

Social Gatherings

I was casually scrolling through an ADHD support group on Facebook the other day when I came across a lady who posted about her mental health deteriorating because of a dinner party that included her in-laws. She went on to state that the planning was incredibly stressful, and that had me thinking.

Social gatherings are stressful situations. Let's face it, a lot of us probably dread them. I guess I don't have them, they just cause unnecessary anxiety over simple things. If you're hosting a dinner party, a birthday party, or any other kind of social gathering, you might need a few tips on how to deal with them, stress-free!

Tips on How to Host and Plan Without Unnecessary Stress!

The first thing that you'll probably do is decide on what kind of event you're planning on hosting. Is it a formal event? Informal? Does it have any kind of theme? The second most important part of your event is the guest list. Are you planning on inviting parents and children? If you're inviting everyone, will your entertainment be child-friendly?

Once you've decided on the type of event it'll be and your guest list, you can go ahead and take a breather. You've just handled the first two steps! Remember to take frequent breaks to ensure that you're not overloading your mind and your emotional state. As a woman with ADHD, it's important to take care of yourself during this kind of planning. Don't overwhelm yourself by trying to do everything in one go. It's helpful to plan further ahead to give yourself more time to plan.

Get Some Help!

Don't be afraid to ask your partner or a friend to help you plan any kind of social event. It doesn't mean that you're not capable of doing it by yourself, it simply means that the task can be done more efficiently and faster if you have some help.

Let's work on a scenario. You're a married woman with three children and you're hosting a dinner party for close friends and family. The total number of guests ended up being around 15 people. Your dinner table might not cut it, so in this case, you could consider hosting the dinner party outside.

You can make it an informal event by throwing some old blankets on the grass and making it a picnic, or you could rent/borrow tables and chairs.

If you really want to make most social gatherings hassle-free, opt for barbeques! Just whip up a few side salads and add some rolls and you've got a meal! If you prefer cooking, your meal will have to be carefully planned.

Firstly, whether you're cooking or throwing something on the grill, you need to consider the dietary needs of your guests. Are there going to be vegans or vegetarians present? Are there any potentially dangerous allergies?

You can make sure of this information by asking your guests to inform you at a certain chosen date before your event. This can give you enough time to plan for every potential scenario.

Meal Planning

Meal prepping for people is a task that is fundamentally undesirable for people with ADHD. In contrast, the inventiveness required to put together a last-minute dinner with whatever is available is ADHD-friendly (albeit meals produced on the fly are unlikely to meet nutritional standards night after night).

If you're struggling with the never-ending need to plan and prepare food, try this ADHD-friendly strategy. These simple meal plans will allow you to breeze through the shopping aisles and have supper on the table in no time!

The Six-Step Meal System

1. Conduct a family meeting. Dinnertime is the ideal time. Inquire with family members about their preferred meal menus. Although children's tastes should be considered, consider the nutritional balance of every meal they offer.

2. Make a "Top-Ten" meal list. You'll prepare these meals well over two weeks, with two nights per week free to order in or eat out.

3. Make individual notecards for your dinner menus, detailing all of the items as well as the ingredients for complicated meals.

4. Arrange your meal notes with a focus on time-saving sequences. If you grill chicken breasts on Monday night, cook a couple extra to slice up and throw into your chicken Caesar salad on Tuesday or Wednesday.

5. Keep the notecards on hand at all times. Keep those in your handbag or wallet, paper-clipped into two groups so you may go shopping anytime you want.

6. Take your notes to the supermarket and you'll have your meals prepared and the majority of your grocery list already written down.

How to Customize the Meal System for Your Family

The virtue of this approach is its adaptability. It's more than simply an ADHD-friendly food plan; it's *your* ADHD-friendly meal plan. Here are a few simple methods for making it work for you:

- Allow "free evenings" to float. Take a free night if an emergency arises or if you simply need a break. Then, the next day, go on to the next note.

- Refresh the menu. If your family becomes tired of the initial top ten dinner meals, call another family gathering to get fresh meal options.

- Be open to new experiences. If something fantastic is on sale, or if you simply have a strong desire to purchase something that's not on your meal plan, go for it! The meal cards aren't intended to limit you; they're there to help you. They'll be waiting for you until you're ready to restart the system.

Four Ways to Make Meal Preparation Even Easier

Keep the following easy concepts in mind as you adopt the ADHD-friendly meal system:

1. Divide your shopping into sections. A once-a-week shopping session can be exhausting and can last the good part of a day. Why not arrange two excursions to the grocery every week, each with two or three meal cards?

2. Share the burden of supper preparations. Each of the five nights of every week, appoint an "assigned cook." Younger children can help the "chef" by preparing the table, collecting ingredients, and so on. Middle and high school students can learn how to make one or two of the top ten family dinners.

They may relish the opportunity to prepare one of their favorite dishes for the rest of the family.

3. Thaw ahead of time. As you make tonight's supper, take out the frozen components for tomorrow night's dinner. In the morning, move them from the counter to the refrigerator. (If you fail to start thawing the night before, you'll have another opportunity in the morning!)

4. Cook in quadruple batches and freeze the extras. Go ahead and do it; you'll have more free nights this way.

Easy Meals

Not every event needs to have a three-course meal or even a dessert! But if you're looking to really make your guests happy, it's best to include a dessert. Who doesn't like cake? I am going to list a few easy starters, main meals, and desserts that won't have you crying in front of the stove for fear of failing!

It could be considered as my worst fear and problem when it comes to hosting this kind of event. What do I feed these people? Well, here are some easy recipes. I did the searching so you don't have to!

Starters

Starters don't have to be fancy or complicated. Most people enjoy a simple and delicious treat, and that makes less work and stress (Dixon, C. n.d.).

Onion Rings

Onion rings are a simple and easy starter to consider. These don't take a lot of time or too much prep.

Prep Time: 15 minutes

Cook Time: 3 minutes

Total Time: 18 minutes

Serves: 3

Ingredients:

- 1 large onion, preferably sliced into rings
- 1 ¼ cups of flour
- 1 teaspoon of baking powder
- 1 teaspoon of salt
- 1 egg
- 1 cup of milk
- ¾ cup of bread crumbs
- oil for frying as needed

Directions:

Heat your oil to around 365 degrees. If you have a fryer, that's great. Otherwise, a deep pot will work just fine.

Mix the baking powder, flour, and salt in a salad bowl or whatever you have that might work.

Try getting all of the onion rings coated with the flour mixture before mixing the egg and milk in along with the other ingredients.

Now, you can dip your onion rings into the mixture and then into the bread crumbs that should be in a separate bowl.

Be sure that the coating sticks and doesn't drip from the onions. You can deep fry them for a few minutes until they look ready to you. Some people prefer them golden brown, others prefer them just done. Whatever works for you.

Season them with whatever you enjoy and store them in a container until your guests arrive. Onion rings are best when they are warm and fresh.

Halloumi with Thyme and Honey

While searching for interesting and easy starter recipes for a dinner party of my own, I came across this one that seems to be very popular on the internet! Halloumi is a personal favorite food of mine, and for those of you who may not know, it's cheese made from goat milk.

Prep Time: 15 minutes

Cook Time: 15 minutes

Total Time: 15 minutes

Serves: 4

Ingredients:

- 8 oz of cut halloumi
- 1 teaspoon oregano (preferably dried)
- 1 teaspoon of chili flakes (preferably dried)
- lemon juice to taste
- 1 garlic clove (finely crushed)
- 2 tablespoons of extra-virgin olive oil
- a palmful of pine nuts

- 1, 1 oz of rocket

- 1½ tablespoon of raw honey

- thyme leaves, about 4 springs

Directions:

Place the halloumi in a crosshatch pattern, about 1 cm wide and 1 cm deep. Don't cut all the way through.

Mix the oregano, chili, and lemon juice, garlic, olive oil, and some black pepper. Marinade the halloumi and spoon it into the crosshatches. Cover the marinated halloumi and store it in the fridge either overnight or at least for a few hours.

Toast the pine nuts over medium heat for no more than 3 minutes. Place the finished product into a bowl and store for later.

Remember to preheat the griddle pan, then grill the halloumi for a few minutes on each side in a bit of olive oil.

You can serve the honey on some rocket or with any other side you prefer, drizzle a little honey over the finished product.

Main Meals

These two main meal ideas are great as stand-alone meals or with starters and desserts. These classic recipes are easy enough for anyone to make and are enjoyable for the whole family (Top 100 easy dinner recipes, 2018).

Lasagna

Prep Time: 20 minutes

Cook Time: 1 hour

Total Time: 1 hour and 20 minutes

Serves: 8

Ingredients:

- 2 teaspoons of olive oil
- 1 brown onion (chopped finely)
- 2 cloves of garlic (chopped)
- 26, 50 oz of beef mince (any kind you prefer, substitute with lentils or soy mince for vegetarian option)
- 2 400g cans of tomatoes (preferably diced, or fresh diced tomatoes)
- 1/2 a cup of dry red wine
- 1/4 cup of tomato paste
- Salt and ground pepper
- Extra olive oil for greasing
- 4 lasagne sheets
- 1/2 cup of coarsely grated Devondale Mozzarella Cheese Block
- Salad leaves for serving
- Cheese sauce
- 4 cups of milk (whichever milk you prefer)
- Another brown onion (chopped coarsely)
- Fresh parsley

- Around 8 peppercorns
- 2 bay leaves
- 2, 12 oz of butter
- 1/3 cup of all-purpose flour (or plain flour)
- 1 cup of parmesan cheese (grated)
- Ground nutmeg (just a pinch)
- Ground white pepper

Any of the above ingredients can be substituted for vegetarian or vegan options if you prefer them.

Heat your oil in a frying pan, preferably a larger one. Don't set the heat too hot; medium heat is preferable. Mix your onion and some garlic and fry it for around 5 minutes to caramelize the onions, then you can add your mince or other options and stir the dish until the mince seems somewhat cooked. You can then add your tomato, wine, and tomato paste and stir for a minute or two before leaving it for another minute until the mixture is brought to a boil.

By this time, you can bring the heat down and let the dish simmer without covering the pan. It should take about 30 minutes for the sauce to thicken and the mince to be cooked thoroughly. You can add the salt and pepper at any time during this stage and add as much or as little as you like. Remember that your guests can add extra salt to their meal, but too much salt cannot be removed after it's been added by the cook (AKA you).

For the cheese sauce, you can add the milk, onion, and parsley together with the peppercorn, cloves, and bay leaves. Place the mixture in a slightly smaller saucepan (although the size doesn't really matter too much) and let it simmer for a few minutes before removing it and letting it sit for about 15 minutes.

The milky mixture can be strained and placed into a jug. Then you can melt your butter in a saucepan until it starts to foam. Slowly add your flour and stir for a minute or two until the mixture starts boiling. At this point, you can remove it from the heat.

Slowly add half of the milk and whisk until smooth, then add the rest of the milk and continue whisking until you're left with a smooth mixture.

Place the saucepan back over the heat until it boils and continue stirring to prevent clots. The sauce needs to be thick and creamy before you remove it from the heat again and add the parmesan cheese. The cheese needs to melt fully into your mixture before you can add more salt, white pepper, and some nutmeg.

Remember to preheat your oven to 356°F. Use a rectangular oven dish and grease it lightly with oil, the oven dish should have at least a 12-cup capacity. Add a quarter of the bechamel sauce to the dish and spread evenly. After you're satisfied with the spread of the sauce, you can arrange a lasagne sheet over it and then place a third of the mince dish over that.

Add a third of the remaining sauce over the mince and then add another lasagne sheet. Continue to layer the rest of the dish in this order and finish it with the last bit of sauce. To top off your lasagne, you can sprinkle the mozzarella cheese over the top. Bake your dish in the oven for about 40 minutes. Be sure to check on your lasagne frequently to prevent it from burning. Trust me, I have had my fair share of burnt lasagne because of my mind wandering off.

After you're satisfied with how cooked the meal is, you can cut it into portions. This recipe was originally made to serve 8, but that depends on how you like your portion sizes. Mixed salad leaves are preferred as a side dish, but I kind of like adding a proper salad to the mix.

Here are the ingredients to my favorite kind of salad:

- Lettuce or mixed leaves

- Feta cheese
- Olives
- Mixed peppers
- Tomatoes (chopped or cherry tomatoes, whatever you prefer)
- Onions (chopped)
- Cucumber (chopped)
- Avo (sliced)
- Pineapple (chopped)
- Blueberries

A salad is a salad, right? You can add any ingredients that you like for the perfect side dish to any main meal, be it a barbeque or a formal dinner.

Chicken and Vegetable Stir Fry

Prep Time: 20 minutes

Cook Time: 10 minutes

Total Time: 30 minutes

Serves: 4

Ingredients:

- 2 tablespoons of peanut oil
- 3 chicken breasts (cut into strips)
- 1 brown onion (cut into thin slices)

- 1 red capsicum (cut into thin slices, no seeds)
- 8,9 oz of button mushrooms (chopped or whole, whichever you prefer)
- Broccolini (chopped or sliced)
- Fresh ginger (chopped)
- 2 cloves of garlic (chopped)
- 2 fresh chilies (chopped with or without seeds)
- 2 tablespoons of soy sauce (preferably salt-reduced)
- 1 1/2 tablespoons of oyster sauce
- 1 tablespoon of clean water
- 3, 6 oz of bean sprouts (to serve with)
- Coriander leaves (also to serve with)
- Cooked rice (white or brown, to serve with)

All of the "to serve with" options are simply options. You can leave them out or substitute them with whatever you like! Some of you might prefer serving a stir fry on its own without any starches, and that's perfectly fine. Others might prefer noodles over rice. You're the cook, you know yourself and your guests. Whatever works!

Directions:

So, you can use a wok (a Chinese type of pan/pot) if you have one, or you can use a large frying pan. Start by heating the wok/pan over high heat for a minute or two and then add a tablespoon of oil to grease the surface. Once it's hot enough, you can add the chicken strips or about half of them, depending on the size of your wok/pan.

It should only take a few minutes for the chicken to cook through. Don't overcook the chicken. Once it's just through, you can remove it and add it to a separate plate or bowl for later.

Next, you can start frying the onions and capsicum in the same wok/pan. It should also only take a few minutes to cook. The mushrooms and broccoli can be added at this point. You can keep stirring for another minute or two and then add the ginger along with the garlic and chilies. You can season the vegetables with salt or any other spices you like.

When you're sure that the vegetables are well cooked, you can add the oyster sauce, the water, and the soy sauce. Add the pre-cooked chicken and stir the dish until the sauces are properly mixed and coating the food.

After you are satisfied with the flavor, you can remove the dish from the heat and add bean sprouts and coriander to give it that fresh touch. Ready to go!

Desserts

You know what? Everyone needs a dessert recipe or two close by. Not just for guests, but for the occasional spoil! These two desserts are personal favorites that never fail to impress the taste buds. Since you might have spent a lot of time cooking to finally get to this part, we'll go with recipes that don't even require baking.

Icebox Cake (Abraham, 2019)

Prep Time: 5 minutes

Cook Time: N/A

Total Time: Around 4 and a half hours

Serves: 8

Ingredients:

- 3 cups of heavy cream
- 1/2 cup of powdered sugar
- 1 teaspoon of vanilla extract
- 64 Oreo thins/wafers
- extra Oreos or wafers for serving

Directions:

Start by mixing the cream, vanilla, and powdered sugar together in a bowl. You can use a hand mixer to beat the ingredients until they form stiff peaks.

Use a springform pan and then simply start layering the ingredients. First the cream and then the cookies. Layer these until you have at least 4 layers of cookies (can be more if you prefer it).

For the final step, you simply refrigerate the cake for around 4 hours or more. There you go! This dessert can be made the evening before your event or get-together.

Peanut Butter Banana Pudding (Abraham, 2018)

This dessert is quite popular. While I was looking for the original recipe, I found that it was a common dessert among internet users. Since this is a peanut butter dessert, you should make sure that none of your guests have any allergies to nuts.

Prep Time: 5 minutes

Cook Time: N/A

Total Time: Around 4 and a half hours

Serves: 8

Ingredients:

- 1 ⅓ cups of milk
- 3.4 oz of ready mix packaged vanilla pudding
- 14 oz of sweetened condensed milk
- 3 cups of heavy cream
- ¼ cups of powdered sugar
- 1 teaspoon of vanilla extract
- 2 cups of melted peanut butter
- 16 oz of "box nutter butters"
- 4 bananas (sliced)

Directions:

Mix the milk, vanilla pudding, and condensed milk together in a big bowl and whisk it thoroughly. Place the mixture in the fridge for 5-10 minutes.

You can then mix the heavy cream with the powdered sugar and vanilla extract. Beat this mixture for about 3 minutes and you'll see stiff peaks forming. Keep about ⅓ of the mixture aside and mix the rest into the first pudding mixture.

Preferably use a trifle dish, but whatever you have is fine. The first layer will be the pudding mixture, then an even layer of cookies. After this, you can layer banana slices. Continue layering the ingredients and then top it off with the mixture that you previously set aside.

This dish can also be made the previous night, as it needs to set in the fridge. If you'd like, you can serve it with crumbled cookies and cream.

What's Next?

The next part is the fun part. If you plan on decorating, you'll need to decide how you'll be decorating the area that you've chosen for your gathering. Get creative! Women with ADHD are known for their creative sides, and this is the perfect opportunity for you to show off your skills.

Whether it's simplistic or fancy, it doesn't matter. As long as it gives your guests a sense of you.

In the end, no woman is expected to handle these events or gatherings alone anymore. Some of us might not even enjoy playing the part of hostess. But if you're like me and you enjoy it, it doesn't need to be a pain in the backside.

You can practice any relaxing techniques before the planning and the get-together itself. This will help you keep calm throughout the process.

Conclusion

At the end of this book begins the start of your new life. Now you understand how precious you are and how not normal but perfectly abnormal we are. In this book, I've outlined some of the advice that I wish could have been given to me in one sitting, instead of me having to go to multiple sources before finding the inspiration that I so desperately needed. I hope that the information in this book will prove useful and helpful to every person who reads it.

My mission is to see that women with ADHD get the help that they need while still accepting themselves for the sentient beings that they are. We deserve love and respect, too, regardless of which conditions we may or may not have.

You're Not Alone!

If there is one bit of information throughout this entire book that I wish would sink in, it is this: You're not alone. I could say it a million times and it would never lose its meaning. For every lonely moment that you might have experienced throughout your life, there is another woman out there who has felt exactly the same.

This doesn't mean that your feelings of loneliness aren't valid or real, it simply means that you can reach out to like-minded people who understand you. There are so many of us once you start looking, and you will never stop finding us. Just as you might be feeling lonely, or as you might have felt before, other women feel the same. For this reason, it's good to reach out to one another and to offer a shoulder.

Along with the relevant social media groups, there are also support groups available online or in-person, depending on your preference or the regulations set in place for the pandemic in your area. Do yourself a favor and look them up. You might be surprised by what you'll learn, or by what you can teach others.

While we stress the fact that there are women who face similar challenges as we do, we also need to acknowledge that every situation is unique. Genetics and the environment play a huge role in how we experience certain symptoms. For this reason, it's also good to pay attention to the women around you. A fresh perspective might just be what you need to motivate yourself.

You Can Overcome Anything That Life Throws at You

With that said, you should remember that regardless of your background or your past mistakes, you can overcome anything that life throws at you. You have so much more power within you than you'll realize at this moment. Hopefully, as you learn and live, your own true worth will become more clear to you.

It doesn't matter if you've lost your temper in the past, or if a job opportunity didn't work out because of your symptoms or other situations. What matters is how you move forward and handle the new challenges that every day will surely bring. If you commit to bettering yourself and to learning as much as you can about your condition, this is more than possible.

Always Remember This!

Your future is in your hands and your hands alone. Another key takeaway of this book was to be sure to always conduct your own research on treatment forms; you never know what new kinds of treatment may be on the horizon. The research you conduct will also ensure that you're comfortable with anything that your doctor suggests. Just keep in mind that while you've conducted extensive research, your doctor spent years studying the very condition that you have. For this reason, their advice is always important and should be taken seriously.

I can't stress enough the importance of taking your medication exactly as prescribed, especially if you're on stimulant medications. These medications can have a highly addictive outcome when taken in uncontrolled doses that could lead to severe health effects. Always consult with your doctor if you aren't sure about your dose or if you've missed a dose. You should never take a double dose if one has been missed.

I also feel like it's important for you to remember that even though you might feel overwhelmed now, you can still manage your symptoms. By referring to some of the tips and advice I've provided you with and by conducting your own research, along with the help of your doctor, nothing is as hopeless as it may seem.

Women are wired differently than men. Some say that this is a myth, but from my own experience, I can say that I believe it. That doesn't mean that men feel less than we do or that they don't deserve as much support as we do, it just means that we're different, and that's okay. We should embrace our differences because where one of us falls short, the other can pick up the pieces.

In a united world, we can all face the obstacles that have been put in our ways, women standing together as one, with men by our sides as our equal companions. Never give up on yourself, never give up on a loved one with this condition, never give up on each other! I hope that I've made a difference for you today, so that you can thrive in your community, wearing your ADHD as a symbol of bravery instead of a badge of failure.

Life can be beautiful, life can be meaningful, and "life could be a dream, sweetheart."

References

ADDitude Editors. (2016, November 29). *What I would never trade away*. ADDitude; ADDitude. https://www.additudemag.com/slideshows/positives-of-adhd/

ADHD Superpowers. (2020, August 12). Minnesota Neuropsychology, LLC. https://www.mnneuropsychology.com/articles/ADHD_Superpowers.html

American Academy of Pediatrics. (2019, September 27). *Causes of ADHD: What We Know Today*. HealthyChildren.org. https://www.healthychildren.org/English/health-issues/conditions/adhd/Pages/Causes-of-ADHD.aspx

Anderson, K. N., Ailes, E. C., Danielson, M., Lind, J. N., Farr, S. L., Broussard, C. S., & Tinker, S. C. (2018). Attention-Deficit/Hyperactivity Disorder Medication Prescription Claims Among Privately Insured Women Aged 15–44 Years — United States, 2003–2015. *MMWR. Morbidity and Mortality Weekly Report*, *67*(2), 66–70. https://doi.org/10.15585/mmwr.mm6702a3

Brain Forest Centers. (2019, September 18). *Everything you need to know about neurofeedback therapy*. Brain Forest. https://www.brainforestcenters.com/news/everything-you-need-to-know-about-neurofeedback-therapy

Carey, M. P., & Forsyth, A. D. (2009). *Self-efficacy teaching tip sheet. Https://Www.apa.org.* https://www.apa.org/pi/aids/resources/education/self-efficacy

Castañeda, S. B. (2016, March 7). *5 Successful women with ADHD who talk about It.* Bustle. https://www.bustle.com/articles/144615-5-successful-women-with-adhd-who-talk-about-it

CHADD. (2018). *Relationships & social skills - CHADD.* CHADD. https://chadd.org/for-adults/relationships-social-skills/

Daniels, L. (2021, January 25). *The benefits of exercise for your physical and mental health.* Www.medicalnewstoday.com. https://www.medicalnewstoday.com/articles/benefits-of-exercise#diabetes

DeBakey, M. E. (2020, October 29). *A perfect match: The health benefits of jigsaw puzzles.* Baylor College of Medicine Blog Network. https://blogs.bcm.edu/2020/10/29/a-perfect-match-the-health-benefits-of-jigsaw-puzzles/#:~:text=Puzzles%20are%20also%20good%20for

Diagnosing ADHD in adults: how adults are tested for ADHD. (2021, January 26). WebMD. https://www.webmd.com/add-adhd/diagnosing-adhd-adults

Dixon, C. (n.d.). *Marinated halloumi with honey and thyme recipe.* Sainsbury`s Magazine. Retrieved December 6, 2021, from https://www.sainsburysmagazine.co.uk/recipes/mains/marinated-halloumi-with-honey-and-thyme

Garrity, A. (2021, May 20). *Modern tips for the tidiest home ever*. Good Housekeeping. https://www.goodhousekeeping.com/home/tips/g2610/best-organizing-tips/

Gunnerson, T. (2020, July 2). *A brief history of ADHD*. WebMD. https://www.webmd.com/add-adhd/adhd-history

Harrar, S. (2016). *ADHD treatments: 5 really promising research updates*. PsyCom.net - Mental Health Treatment Resource since 1986. https://www.psycom.net/adhd-treatments-research

Head, A. (2021, September 14). *Self care ideas: 27 totally free ways to practice self-care*. Marie Claire. https://www.marieclaire.co.uk/life/health-fitness/self-care-ideas-725076

Healthwise Staff. (2020, January 30). *ADHD Myths and facts*. Wa.kaiserpermanente.org. https://wa.kaiserpermanente.org/kbase/topic.jhtml?docId=hw164660

Holland, K. (2015, February 26). *The history of ADHD: a timeline*. Healthline; Healthline Media. https://www.healthline.com/health/adhd/history#1902

How the gender gap leaves girls and women undertreated for ADHD. (n.d.). CHADD. https://chadd.org/adhd-news/adhd-news-caregivers/how-the-gender-gap-leaves-girls-and-women-undertreated-for-adhd/

How to declutter your home: a ridiculously thorough guide. (n.d.). Www.budgetdumpster.com. https://www.budgetdumpster.com/resources/how-to-declutter-your-home.php

Hurley, K. (2016). *ADHD in the workplace - tips to flourish in the work environment.* Psycom.net - Mental Health Treatment Resource since 1986. https://www.psycom.net/adhd-in-the-workplace/

Katzman, M. A., Bilkey, T. S., Chokka, P. R., Fallu, A., & Klassen, L. J. (2017). Adult ADHD and comorbid disorders: clinical implications of a dimensional approach. *BMC Psychiatry, 17*(1). https://doi.org/10.1186/s12888-017-1463-3

Kinman, T. (2016, March 22). *Gender differences in ADHD symptoms.* Healthline; Healthline Media. https://www.healthline.com/health/adhd/adhd-symptoms-in-girls-and-boys#ADHD-and-Gender-

Littman, E. (2018, January 29). *Women with ADHD: no more suffering in silence.* ADDitude. https://www.additudemag.com/gender-differences-in-adhd-women-vs-men/

Louw, K. (2019). *Why many women with ADHD remain undiagnosed.* Verywell Mind. https://www.verywellmind.com/add-symptoms-in-women-20394

Louw, K. (2019, November 22). *7 Types of ADD you should know about.* Verywell Mind. https://www.verywellmind.com/understanding-dr-daniel-amens-6-types-of-add-20466

Martin, J. (2014, January 23). *ADHD and the importance of healthy sleep.* National Elf Service. https://www.nationalelfservice.net/mental-health/sleep-disorders/adhd-and-the-importance-of-healthy-sleep/

Morin, A. (n.d.). *8 common myths about ADHD.* Www.understood.org. https://www.understood.org/articles/en/common-myths-about-adhd

NHS Choices. (2019). *Causes - Attention deficit hyperactivity disorder (ADHD).* NHS. https://www.nhs.uk/conditions/attention-deficit-hyperactivity-disorder-adhd/causes/

Parekh, R. (2017, July). *What is ADHD?* Psychiatry.org; American Psychiatric Association. https://www.psychiatry.org/patients-families/adhd/what-is-adhd

Park, S. (2019, May 25). *Famous women with ADHD.* POPSUGAR Fitness. https://www.popsugar.com/fitness/photo-gallery/46084806/image/46094340/Margaux-Joffe

Posner, J. (2006, October 6). *9 ADHD myths and fallacies that perpetuate stigma.* ADDitude. https://www.additudemag.com/adhd-myths-and-facts-learn-the-truth-about-attention-deficit/

Raypole, C. (2019, September 3). *How to improve concentration: 12 science-backed tips, and more.* Healthline. https://www.healthline.com/health/mental-health/how-to-improve-concentration#brain-training

Raypole, C. (2020, April 28). *How to control your emotions: 11 strategies to try.* Healthline. https://www.healthline.com/health/how-to-control-your-emotions#consider-the-impact

Rodden, J. (2019, July 2). *The history of ADHD and its treatments.* ADDitude. https://www.additudemag.com/history-of-adhd/

Roth, E., & Weiss, K. (2013). *What are the three types of ADHD?* Healthline. https://www.healthline.com/health/adhd/three-types-adhd

Rucklidge, J. J. (2010). Gender differences in attention-deficit/hyperactivity disorder. *The Psychiatric Clinics of North America, 33*(2), 357–373. https://doi.org/10.1016/j.psc.2010.01.006

Seay, B. (2006, October 6). *Supermom Is overrated!* ADDitude. https://www.additudemag.com/parenting-moms-with-adhd-advice-help/

Semeco, A. (2017, February 10). *The top 10 benefits of regular exercise.* Healthline. https://www.healthline.com/nutrition/10-benefits-of-exercise#TOC_TITLE_HDR_2

Sherrell, Z. (2021, July 21). *What are the benefits of ADHD?* Www.medicalnewstoday.com. https://www.medicalnewstoday.com/articles/adhd-benefits

Smith, M. (2019). *Adult ADHD and relationships.* HelpGuide.org. https://www.helpguide.org/articles/add-adhd/adult-adhd-attention-deficit-disorder-and-relationships.htm

Taylor, J., & Ph.D. (2008, July 18). *13 Survival strategies for moms with ADHD.* ADDitude. https://www.additudemag.com/when-moms-have-adhd-too/

Voge, D. (2019). *Understanding and overcoming procrastination | McGraw Center for Teaching and Learning.* Princeton.edu. https://mcgraw.princeton.edu/understanding-and-overcoming-procrastination

Watson, S. (2012, May 31). *Adult ADHD and exercise.* WebMD; WebMD. https://www.webmd.com/add-adhd/adult-adhd-and-exercise

Williamson, E. (2021, May 18). *Mental health disorder.* The Emma Williamson. https://theemmawilliamson.com/the-gray-block/mental-health-disorder-2/

Abraham, L. (2018, March 6). *Peanut butter lovers will DIE over this Peanut Butter Banana Pudding.* Delish. https://www.delish.com/cooking/recipe-ideas/recipes/a58604/peanut-butter-banana-pudding-recipe/

Abraham, L. (2019, May 28). *This magical icebox cake has only 4 ingredients*. Delish. https://www.delish.com/cooking/recipe-ideas/a27469997/icebox-cake-recipe/

Silver, L. (2011, April 18). *ADHD or ADD medications for adults and children: Stimulants, nonstimulants & More*. ADDitude. https://www.additudemag.com/adhd-medication-for-adults-and-children/

Top 100 easy dinner recipes. (2018, August 29). Www.taste.com.au. https://www.taste.com.au/quick-easy/galleries/top-100-easy-dinner-recipes/biccuul7

Manufactured by Amazon.ca
Bolton, ON